BACK IN CONTROL!

BACK IN CONTROL!

A Conventional and Complementary Prescription for Eliminating Back Pain

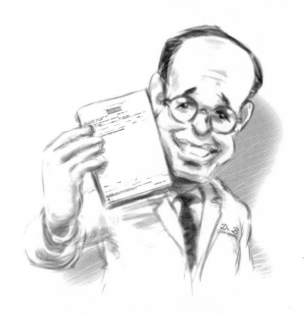

DAVID BORENSTEIN, M.D.

M. Evans and Company, Inc.
New York

M. Evans and Company, Inc.
216 East 49th Street
New York, New York 10017

Library of Congress Cataloging-in-Publication Data

Borenstein, David G.
    Back in control! : conventional and complementary prescription for relieving back pain / by David Borenstein
        p.   cm.
    ISBN 0-87131-945-4
    1. Backache 2. Backache—Alternative treatment. I. Title
RD771.V217 B669 2001
617.5'64—dc21   2001023344

Book design and typesetting by Evan H. Johnston

Printed in the United States of America

9   8   7   6   5   4   3   2   1

ATTENTION:

This book includes the most up-to-date information about conventional and complementary therapy for low back pain, based upon my twenty-two years of clinical experience with people with spine problems. The object of this book is to educate people about low back pain and offer relief of this disorder. Despite these good intentions, this book cannot offer any guarantee about the ultimate resolution of your back condition. Do not be tempted to use this book as a substitute for a medical evaluation. An examination by a health professional is always an appropriate approach to the evaluation of low back pain. Your physician has the unique advantage of listening to your description of your problem and completing a physical examination before forming an opinion about your back pain. The information in this book may differ from the advice offered by your health care provider. The recommendations in this book are not meant to replace medical treatment or diagnosis by your physician. When in doubt about the advice you have received, obtain a second opinion from another health care professional. Ultimately, you are solely responsible for your own medical decisions.

This book is dedicated to all my patients who have given me the honor of being their physician. This work is the result of their persistent requests to put my explanations of their back problems on paper.

CONTENTS

PART TWO: KNOWING YOUR TREATMENT OPTIONS

PART THREE: LIVING WITHOUT BACK PAIN

ACKNOWLEDGMENTS

I want to thank the individuals who have been willing to lend support, encouragement, and expertise in the development and review of this book:

Arthur Frank, M.D., medical director of the Weight Management program at the George Washington University Medical Center, for his thoughtful comments concerning the food and nutrition sections of this book.

John Starr, M.D., orthopaedic surgeon, for offering his expertise in reviewing the surgical components of this book.

Tom Welsh, R.P.T., physical therapist, for his generosity and friendship in allowing his exercise program to be included in this book.

Virginia McCullough, for organizing my first manuscript proposal, finding my book agent, and helping me with my first draft.

Marian Betancourt, for helping me with my final draft of this book.

Nancy Love, my literary agent, for having confidence in me and finding a company to publish my book.

Judy Guenther, illustrator, for taking my ideas and drawing illustrations that make understanding much easier.

PJ Dempsey, my editor at M. Evans, for guiding me through the beginning, middle, and end of a very long process that has resulted in the publication of this book.

My partners at Arthritis and Rheumatism Associates—John Lawson, M.D.; Werner Barth, M.D.; Norman Koval, M.D.; Herbert Baraf, M.D.; Robert Rosenberg, M.D.; Evan Siegel, M.D.; Emma DiIorio, M.D.; and Sheila Kelly, M.D.—for being supportive and understanding during the development and production of this book.

INTRODUCTION

ONE BIG SNEEZE CAN DO YOU IN

I knew better than to bend over to grab a pair of socks from the bottom drawer—that was my first mistake. I knew I should bend my knees and reach down, rather than bending "in half." Twisting from the waist was my second mistake, although I had used that motion thousands of times and it had never affected me the way it did now. Just as I started to straighten up, I felt a sharp pain on the right side of my back as the muscles there went into spasm. The pain was like a knife cut—it literally took my breath away, and I couldn't move.

Rational thinking and severe pain do not go hand in hand. In fact, when one is in pain, the most ridiculous thoughts seem perfectly reasonable. Bracing myself against the dresser that morning, I began to consider how I would put my clothes on without feeling the excruciating pain in my back. The socks in my hands seemed miles away from my feet, so how would I ever get them on? Limping as I put one foot in front of the other, bracing against the furniture for support, I began to gather up other clothes, being careful to test each small motion to see if it would bring on more pain. Putting on my shirt wasn't so bad, but I couldn't imagine how I would get my pants on. So, maybe I could just show up at the office without them. Perhaps the staff wouldn't even notice!

I felt like a prisoner in my body, stuck in one place, in one position. I tried to straighten up a couple of times before I was successful, but my back was stiff and it took great effort. As if I didn't have enough going on, a big sneeze "exploded" before I could prevent it—and the spontaneous body movements that came with it. I had thought my pain was a 10 on a ten-point scale, but I was wrong. The sneeze shot me up to 14 or 15 for at least a few seconds. In addition to the increased intensity of the pain, it was now spreading up and down my back. After the second sneeze, I thought I was going to die.

Eventually, I managed to work up the courage to complete a series of "bracing and bending" movements, and carefully using the handrail on the stairway, I limped down to face breakfast, which I ate standing up. Then I took a couple of pain relievers, hoping that as the day continued my range of motion would improve. Bending over the sink to brush my teeth was out of the question, so I accomplished that task with a towel around my collar and a plastic cup of water.

Driving to my office wasn't so bad—once I had eased myself into the car. As I drove along, I did my best to avoid potholes, which looked deeper than ever. So far, every small decision, every normally routine and insignificant task, required careful consideration. Pain and restricted motion led me to park the car in a place where no neighboring cars would limit how far I could swing my door open, because it would be a chore to get out of the car. With my back straight, I moved my legs around and held on while I stood up. Normally, I get some extra exercise by walking up the stairs to my office, but today, the elevator looked very inviting.

Pain turned my usually comfortable office into a minefield. I had to maneuver around chairs and file cabinets and desks. And the biggest mine in the field was, of all things, my soft cushion recliner. I knew a firmer chair with less give was a much better choice. Throughout the day I continued to make one small choice after another to accommodate the pain and discomfort. For example, I avoided twisting my body to see the computer screen, I carried only two files at a time, and I changed position often in order to avoid becoming stuck in one place. It goes without saying that I canceled my scheduled exercise session with my workout partner.

Pain relievers helped dull the pain throughout the day, and I was able to see my patients without outwardly looking like a patient myself. But all my "extra" tasks—article research, notes to patients or doctors, letters to sign, and so forth—were put aside for another day. There is nothing like back pain to put one's priorities in place.

Even though it took longer, I took a route home that seemed "safer," because it had fewer obstacles and potholes. All this concern and conscious thought about my pain and moving my body was exhausting. Pain is a major stressor, and I wasn't surprised that I was so tired. Eating dinner hardly seemed worth the effort, but if I wanted to take more painkillers, and I did, then I needed to eat.

Standing in the shower and letting the hot water run down my back for a few minutes allowed me to carefully bend and stretch the muscles, which restored some range of motion. I moved slowly, letting the pain guide how far I could bend. This experiment in motion didn't last long, and I didn't move very far, but I would try again tomorrow.

Sleep is always a concern when one is in pain. Getting into bed, which involved lowering my upper back with the help of my arms while at the same time raising my legs, triggered more shots of pain. But at least I was there. I stayed on my back and bent my knees over a pillow. As I drifted off to sleep, I tried to remember what got me into this fix in the first place. Of course— the blasted socks!

Back pain will ruin any day, and it has certainly ruined a few of mine. That's why I wrote this book; not only because I've been treating my patients for back pain, but because my own pain has given me the kinds of insights that helped me develop my basic back pain relief program.

Every second, two Americans develop low back pain. Each year 50 million of us suffer episodes of low back pain. If you are reading this book, you have experienced back pain—you may be in pain right now. Low back pain can begin with something as seemingly trivial as a sneeze, a cough, a simple twisting motion, or even bending over to grab a pair of socks. Or it can be a symptom of a more serious disease.

The men and women who arrive in my office have diverse backgrounds, careers, and lifestyles, but they all share a common complaint. They have sore, aching backs, and the pain almost always interferes with their lives. These patients have something else in common. To one degree or another, they are afraid. Most people are misinformed about both the causes of their pain and the treatments available to solve their problems. This lack of information feeds the fear that hinders recovery. Some people are afraid that they will be unable to work, while others fear their pain is a symptom of a dread disease such as cancer. Some women are concerned about their ability to carry a pregnancy; others want to prevent the progression of a spinal deformity that occurred in a close relative.

Almost all my patients arrive with questions. What can they do to improve their condition? Should they exercise? Will yoga or Tai chi help? Would manipulation "straighten" a crooked spine, relieve musculoskeletal pain, and, best of all, leave them pain-free?

The best way to read this book is from the beginning, because the more

Introduction

you know about how your back works and the reasons why it hurts, the easier it will be to correctly diagnose and relieve your pain. You will learn how to tell whether your pain is mechanical or medical; that is, related to a problem with the dynamics of your musculoskeletal system, or related to a systemic cause like nerve damage from diabetes. I will show you how my basic back pain relief program can help most back pain; how you can work with your doctor to correctly diagnose and treat back pain; and how and when to use drugs, exercise, and even complementary therapies such as relaxation techniques.

Many people let back pain prevent them from doing the things they love, and this is one of the saddest results of back pain. With my book you will learn how to get into and out of bed without hurting your back, and also— and very important—how to enjoy sex without hurting your back. In the back of the book you will find many resources for more information, as well as my Back School FAQ, which comes from the questions my patients most frequently ask me.

But the most important message I can bring you is that you are in control. The more you learn about how your back works and why it hurts, the better your chances at finding relief from pain. When people don't follow through with a doctor's prescription for their pain, it is most often because they don't really understand how the remedy is supposed to work, or how their body works. I hope this book will help you develop your own unique prescription for back pain relief, and put you back in control.

Now, I am going to take my own advice and put my socks in the top dresser drawer.

PART ONE:
TAKING THE MYSTERY OUT OF LOW BACK PAIN

I

UNDERSTANDING WHY YOUR BACK HURTS

When your back hurts, you feel quite alone. You think that no one can understand the extent of your discomfort. However, low back pain is the second most common affliction of humankind; only the common cold affects more people. Back pain doesn't discriminate, either. People of all ages, both sexes, and all walks of life are afflicted with this debilitating discomfort. Perhaps you are a computer operator who sits at a desk for hours at a time, or maybe you're a farmer or construction worker who engages in heavy lifting every day. If you happen to be a pregnant woman, then you may have difficulty finding any comfortable position—standing or sitting or lying flat on your back.

If you lift, bend, reach, squat, twist, or turn—or even sneeze—you are at some risk for developing back pain. In addition, a variety of medical conditions can result in back pain. So, as you can see, all six or so billion of us are vulnerable to back pain. In fact, it is documented that almost 80 percent of the human population will experience back pain at some point in their lives.

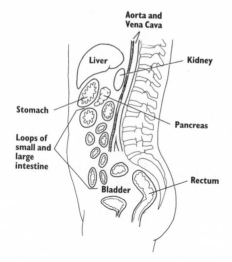

Aorta and Vena Cava

Liver

Kidney

Stomach

Pancreas

Loops of small and large intestine

Rectum

Bladder

Figure 1.1 This side view shows the major organs and blood vessels near the lumbar spine.

IS IT MECHANICAL OR MEDICAL?

Most low back pain results from mechanical disorders of the spine related to overuse, such as habitually poor posture, or injury or deformity of a portion of the spine, such as herniated disc. The other 10 to 15 percent of cases are medical, caused by systemic illnesses such as nerve damage from diabetes or fibromyalgia, and require a more complete evaluation. I refer to this form of back pain as medical low back pain.

Discomfort associated with specific causes of low back pain has reproducible characteristics. For instance, ruptured discs pressing on nerves cause pain that runs from the back to the lower leg and foot. The pain from muscle injuries in the back may spread across the low back but not lower than the buttock. Knowing where the pain initially starts and ends helps us make a good guess about the cause.

Mechanical disorders are caused by local problems in the bones, joints, tendons, ligaments, muscles, and nerves of the low back. Characteristically, being active or at rest has an effect on the intensity of the pain, either making it better or worse. The position of the spine also affects the degree of pain. If you have a disc herniation, you feel more pain when you sit, while people with spinal arthritis feel worse when standing. Most mechanical problems heal or improve with time, physical therapy, and medications. Only 1 to 2 percent of these mechanical difficulties call for surgical intervention, such as when they cause loss of bladder control or leg weakness.

Medical disorders cause symptoms throughout the body and are not limited to discomfort in the lumbar spine, and they don't get better or worse with activity or rest. In addition, many organs such as the kidneys, bladder, gastrointestinal system, lymph nodes, and major blood vessels fit up against the lower back (see fig. 1.1). Diseases that affect these organs can cause back pain, with each organ system causing a certain kind of pain. When back pain originates in a structure other than the spine, the unique character of the pain can help doctors find the diseased organ system.

Medical disorders generally produce these "red flags":

• Fever and/or weight loss
• Pain that is worse at night or when lying down
• Prolonged morning stiffness lasting hours
• Severe bone pain in the middle of the back
• Pain associated with eating, urination, or the menstrual cycle

If you have any of these symptoms, see your doctor to find out if a systemic illness is causing your low back pain.

And while trauma to your back is mechanical, there are times when it becomes an emergency. Direct trauma to the lumbar spine may cause pain in any location in the low back, lower leg, or anterior thigh. These traumas are frequently the result of automobile accidents or falls. If the trauma is severe, emergency surgery may be needed to stabilize the spine and remove pressure on the nerves. Fractures of vertebrae without nerve compression generally call for bracing and rest. Lesser traumas to muscles and ligaments may be treated with medications and physical therapy.

Mary is an example of how medical and mechanical causes of back pain can be confused. Mary loved to work in her garden; and although at sixty-five she had occasional aches and pains after a long day of weeding and pruning, her discomfort disappeared in a day or two. However, one day she tripped and fell backward, landing on her behind. The fall caused acute discomfort that she brushed off at the time, but over the following three weeks the pain in the middle of her back increased in intensity, making it increasingly difficult to work in her garden. When she came to see me, Mary still believed her pain was related to an injury sustained in her fall, but the location and persistence of her pain—in the middle of her back—was a red flag. Her X ray showed a fracture in one of her vertebrae, and blood tests revealed elevation of blood proteins, consistent with a diagnosis of multiple myeloma, a bone marrow cancer. Obviously, her condition called for immediate medical intervention, and she went on to receive a course of chemotherapy. Her back pain improved when the cancer was diagnosed and appropriately treated. While Mary's case clearly falls into the small percentage of cases in which the pain is caused by a medical disorder, her condition calls attention to the importance of addressing pain that does not subside or pain that worsens over time.

Rare Psychological Causes

Psychological or mental illness is a relatively rare cause of acute low back pain. Depending on individual characteristics, psychologic illnesses cause or exacerbate pain through a variety of mechanisms. For example, in schizophrenic patients, hallucinations are a rare but real cause of pain.

The psychiatric disorder commonly associated with low back pain is a conversion reaction: a mechanism for transforming anxiety or other emotions into a physical dysfunction. The symptoms lessen anxiety and symbolize the underlying conflict. Sufferers may benefit from their situation and may not be overly concerned about the physical problem. An abnormal body function, like back pain, is readily recognized and acceptable, but the perception is that psychological problems are not so easily accepted.

Someone with conversion reactions may have severe pain of a burning or cutting quality. The pain is excruciating in intensity and without any recognizable anatomic boundaries. On examination, they have a marked response to minimal pressure on palpation. Their areas of tenderness do not correspond to the tender points of fibromyalgia. Laboratory test results are normal, and in these patients, complaints are resistant to all forms of therapy. Unfortunately, even when the reason for the conversion reaction is evident, these patients may not improve.

The International Association for the Study of Pain defines pain as "an unpleasant sensory and emotional experience which we primarily associate with tissue damage or describe in terms of such damage, or both." The definition of pain has two parts. One part deals with tissue damage or the threat of damage, but to experience pain one must have an emotional response to that injury. Mental stress may elicit an emotional response that is experienced as pain.

HOW YOUR BACK WORKS

After more than twenty years of caring for people with back pain, I've learned that taking the time to explain the anatomy and biomechanics of the lumbar spine goes a long way in helping people understand their situation and alleviate anxiety and fear.

Because most people have no idea of what caused their back injury in the first place, they often experience the same injuries again and again. On the other hand, I've seen people become so afraid of bringing on more pain, even with normal body motion, that they become stiff—like statues. They do not realize that their rigid posture does not protect them from pain, but perpetuates it.

People who don't understand the cause of their pain often do not understand the prescribed treatments, and they don't follow through with self-care, including the specific exercises they are told to perform daily. So, understanding how your back works will help you get rid of pain.

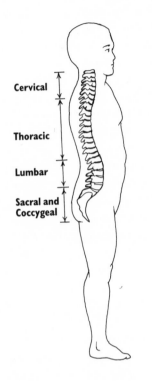

Cervical

Thoracic

Lumbar

Sacral and
Coccygeal

The Lumbar Discs and Bony Joints

The lumbar spine is a beautifully engineered structure with two primary functions: movement and protection of the spinal cord. It is made up of bone, discs, ligaments, muscles, nerves, and blood vessels. The spine contains thirty-three vertebrae, each lined up one atop another and divided into five areas: cervical (neck), thoracic (chest), lumbar (low back), sacral (pelvis), and coccygeal (tail bone).

- Cervical vertebrae facilitate motion in all directions.
- Thoracic vertebrae support the ribs and allow rotation of the body.
- Lumbar vertebrae support the upper part of the body and allow forward and backward motion.
- The sacrum acts as the anchor of the spine and fits between the pelvic bones.

Figure 1.2 From the side you can see how the curves of your spine work to keep your body balanced so your head is directly over over the center of gravity in your pelvis. Notice the balance between the forward curves(lordosis) of the neck and low back and the backward curves(kyphosis) of the chest and pelvis.

When we look at the spine from the side, we can see that it is not straight, but curved. The neck and low back have forward-facing curves, while the chest and sacral spine have backward-facing curves (fig 1.2). These curves allow room for the heart and lungs in the chest, while keeping the head centered over the lower body and the pelvis. This position is well balanced and strong.

Because each section of the spine serves a different function and motion, the vertebrae in each portion of the spine have specific shapes. The lumbar spine contains five vertebrae numbered one through five. You may hear a doctor refer to one of your vertebrae as L-4, for example. This refers to the fourth lumbar vertebra. The assigned letters correspond to the section of the spine.

Facet Joints. Joints are formed where vertebrae meet at top and bottom. Each vertebra has four facet joints, two formed with each vertebra directly above and below, right and left. The vertical orientation allows for bending forward, the greatest degree of motion, and backward, a lesser degree of motion. The structure and orientation of the lumbar facet joints limit the twisting motions of the lumbar spine. The greatest rotation of your spine occurs in the chest, the thoracic portion. The facet joints have cartilage on their surfaces, lining tissue (synovium) that makes joint fluid, and a joint covering, a capsule that keeps the joint fluid in and the bones together.

The "His and Hers" Sacroiliac. The sacrum is a large triangular bone formed by five fused vertebrae wedged between the pelvic bones. The top of the sacrum is the first sacral vertebra, or S-1. The sacroiliac joints are formed between the sacrum and the iliac bones. In this part of the spine, we can see male and female anatomical differences. In men, more of the sacrum is attached to the ilium, and in women, the sacroiliac joints widen during childbirth. These differences also play a role in the typical gait we associate with men and women. In men, the hip structure tends to be stable during normal walking movements; in women there is a natural sway of the hips. The sacrum contains the end of the spinal canal and, therefore, nerves.

The Coccyx. The tail bone, as the coccyx is also known, consists of four tiny fused vertebrae located between the cheeks of the buttocks. This is well padded, which makes it difficult to fracture.

Why You Are Taller in the Morning: Discs Are Cushions and Spacers

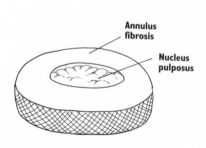

Annulus fibrosis

Nucleus pulposus

The intervertebral discs are the cushions between the vertebral bodies (bones) and make up about one third of the entire height of the lumbar spine. The discs work like universal joints, allowing motion in a number of directions. If vertebral bodies were in direct contact with each other, range of motion would be severely limited.

The disc resembles an automobile tire with a strong balloon filled with a thick gel in the center, where the hub would be in a tire (fig. 1.3). The outer portion of the tire is the annulus fibrosus, layers of fiber that contract or

Figure 1.3 The spinal disc looks much like an automobile tire, with a gel-like center surrounded by a fibrous outer circle.

expand, much like a Chinese finger trap. As we age, the restraining fibers break, and the ability to contain the gel at the center of the disc is compromised or weakened. If the gel moves beyond the boundary of the annulus fibrosus, we have an injury known as a herniated disc, often inaccurately called a slipped disc.

The gel portion of the disc can move forward or backward within the constraints of the "outer tire." The gel moves in opposition to the motion of the spine: forward motion of the spine moves the gel into the back portion of the disc; backward motion does the opposite. The gel can also move side to side. In addition to its ability to facilitate motion, the gel serves as a tremendous shock absorber. If the discs were structured without built-in shock absorbers, our bones would register the full impact of every step we take, and we would have a constant and awful headache.

A disc's cushioning ability depends upon how well the gel remains filled with water. At birth, 88 percent of the gel is water, but this changes as we age. It also changes during the course of the day. At night when there is no pressure on the discs, the gel swells, and we are taller in the morning. As we stand during our waking hours, the weight of the body compresses the discs, making them lose water, and by the end of the day, we are actually shorter. The fact that discs are "fatter" in the morning has some implications for the best time to exercise. As we grow older, the gel in the discs loses water and becomes more easily damaged by daily activities.

The discs not only allow motion between vertebrae, but also act as spacers between the bones. If you look at two vertebrae and a disc from the side (fig. 1.4), you will see a hole, or foramen, between the pedicles above and below the disc in front and the facet joint in back. This allows the nerves to exit the spine to supply other parts of the body. Any disease process that closes the hole has the potential to cause significant back and leg pain by pressing on the exiting nerves.

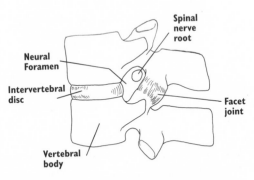

Figure 1.4 This side view of two vertebrae and a disc shows how the spinal bones fit together to protect the nerve root. The opening, called the neural foramen, allows the nerve roots to pass through the spine. Disc damage (herniation) or facet joint degeneration (bone spurs) may narrow the neural foramen, causing compression of the spinal nerve root and resulting in back or leg pain.

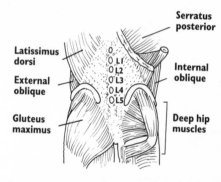

Latissimus dorsi

External oblique

Gluteus maximus

Serratus posterior

Internal oblique

Deep hip muscles

Figure 1.5 Looking at the lumbar spine from the back, you can see the superficial low back muscles on the left and the deeper muscles on the right.

Ligaments Are Like Rubber Bands

Ligaments are strong bands of tissue that act like a girdle or brace around the spine. Both front and back ligaments are closely attached to the outside surfaces of the bone and disc. This "outside packaging" helps keep the parts of the spine in the correct position. The posterior longitudinal ligament (PLL) covers the back of the vertebral bodies from your head to your pelvis and forms the front surface of the spinal canal. It narrows as it passes down the spine and is half its original width by the time it reaches the lumbar spine, and its ability to support discs is weakened. This is why the lumbar area is where disc injury is most likely to occur.

There are other spinal ligaments and all improve stability and restrain excessive movement of the spine. The ligaments act like strong, thick rubber bands, with some give but not too much. Their function is to lend support while limiting motion. The ligaments with more elastic fibers move farther than those without them. As part of the mechanism to accommodate childbirth, women have more elastic fibers than men. In both sexes, all these structures lose elasticity and become stiff with age, which is one reason we lose motion as the years accumulate.

Back Muscles Are Not Our Strongest

Back muscles are among the weakest muscles for the kind of work they are called upon to do, but they play an essential role in the movement of the lumbar spine, as well as in maintaining normal posture (fig. 1.5). A number of muscles in the front of the abdomen and surrounding the spine also

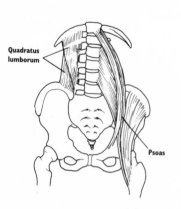

Quadratus lumborum

Psoas

Figure 1.6 This view of the lumbar spine allows you to see how your muscles help the spine move. You can bend forward with the help of the psoas muscle and to the side with the quadratus lumborum.

play a role in both balancing and moving the low back. The largest, but not necessarily the strongest, muscle runs from the base of the skull to the sacrum. This muscle pulls the spine backward and to one side. Smaller muscles allow the spine to bend to the side and perform twisting motions. The *psoas* is a strong muscle that connects the low back with the thigh (fig. 1.6).

Although not officially part of the low back, muscles in the front and sides of the abdomen, the buttocks, the thighs, the hamstrings, and calves all play a role in balancing the spine. The abdominal muscles, including the *rectus abdominus*—the muscle that looks like two columns of rectangles on the front of body builders—have two major purposes. They bend the spine forward, and they also push the organs of the abdomen against the front of the spine, thereby lending it support. Muscles in the buttocks, thighs, and hamstrings need to be flexible to allow rotation around the hips. If these muscles are stiff, normal motion of the spine is limited, which may then result in low back pain.

All the muscles of your lower back are covered with fascia, a membrane that resembles plastic wrap. It surrounds individual muscles and connects them to neighboring muscles. A layer of fascia runs over a major portion of the lumbar spine, just below the skin. This "plastic wrap" enclosure improves the function of the contracting muscles, and while resiliant, it does not contract as muscles do. Fascial tissue is supplied with nerves, and if it stretches or tears, with or without damage to the underlying muscle, it may cause pain.

Nerves: Your Body's Pain Communication System

The role of the nervous system in low back pain is particularly complex because the nervous system itself is so amazing, far more complex than any computer software. However, basic knowledge of the anatomy of the nervous system is essential to understanding the specific pain patterns associated with back pain.

The spinal cord is the major nerve in the spinal canal, and it is constantly sending messages back and forth from the brain to various parts of the body. Moving your big toe, for example, starts with electrical signals that are relayed down the motor nerve column of your spinal cord and through the muscle in your lower leg that lifts your toe. Signals from sensory nerves in your big toe go back up the same nerve through a different sensory column in your spinal cord and report to your brain that the job has been accomplished. Your toe moved.

The spinal cord also has reflexive or involuntary functions, which are controlled by a single level in the spinal cord and do not require intervention from the brain. Let's say your big toe bumps into a rock. The sensory pain

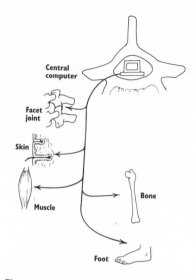

Central computer

Facet joint

Skin

Muscle

Bone

Foot

Figure 1.7 A spinal nerve as a computer network. An injury in one part of the system may affect the network at a distance from the main computer.

nerves send a signal to the sensory column in your spinal cord to report an injury. Your sensory nerve sends a signal to move to the motor nerve at the same level in your spinal cord. Then, through reflexive action, your foot quickly withdraws from pain.

Under normal conditions, you cannot measure the time between the bump and withdrawal because the entire sequence is faster than the split second it takes to mutter "ouch." This reflex requires that the sensory and motor nerves work together at a single level of the spinal cord. If a spinal nerve is compressed near the spinal canal, the reflex associated with that nerve may not work.

The nerve root, as mentioned, passes through a hole in the vertebra—the foramen—and occupies a third of the available space. The rest of the space contains blood vessels, connective tissue, and the sensory nerve for the spine itself, the sinuvertebral nerve. Sensory and muscle functions are separated in the nerve root, and the sensory fibers are affected first when a nerve is compressed. This is why you feel pain before you lose strength. The L-5 is the largest nerve root and is housed in the smallest lumbar foramen, so it is the most vulnerable to compression.

Nerve signals are interconnected with others and spread everywhere, making it hard to find the exact source of pain. Pain travels. Picture the nerves as the cables of a computer network that coordinate function and sensation (fig. 1.7). A single spinal nerve supplies the facet joint, the muscles and skin over the back, and the muscles, bone, and skin of the leg. When the nerve is irritated near the neural foramen, a signal is sent down the nerve reporting an injury. Any structure on that network, even though it is not damaged, may hurt in response to the injury at the level of the spine. An unpleasant sensation experienced away from the original location of injury is called referred pain. People who suffer from back pain and related symptoms are often surprised that their spine is actually the source of numbness in their foot, for example.

HOW YOUR PAIN THRESHOLD FLUCTUATES

If you are under increasing levels of stress, you will be more sensitive to pain. Your pain threshold will be lower. Let's say you stub your big toe with the same force on a Monday morning and a Friday afternoon. On Monday you are rested after an enjoyable weekend. You had a wonderful time and feel well. Your stubbed toe does not hurt very much at all. On Friday, you are exhausted from all the decisions you made during the week. The service people have not come to fix the fax machine, two of the staff are out with the flu, and the deadline for the project is next week. Stress is your middle name. You stub your toe on your desk and you think your foot is going to fall off. The pain is intense. The same amount of injury is felt with a different intensity of pain.

Pain signals to the brain and their perception as pain can be modified by a number of mechanisms. Acupuncture, massage, transcutaneous electrical nerve stimulation (TENS), or surface magnets held by velcro wraps are a few examples of therapies that put sensations into the nervous system to modify signals that are different than the slow pain signals. We'll get to these later in the book.

Another mechanism that blocks pain is the body's production of its own pain relievers, endorphins. These chemicals attach to narcotics receptors in the nerve pathways that block the transmission of pain signals. The release of these endorphins can be accomplished in a number of ways, such as regular exercise. A positive outlook and a reduction of stress can also release endorphins. The belief that a good outcome will be the result of an interaction can have beneficial effects on the healing process, partly mediated through the release of endorphins.

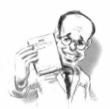

DR. B'S PRESCRIPTION SUMMARY

Rx

- **90 percent of back pain is mechanical in origin.**

- **Mechanical back pain is secondary to overuse or aging.**

- **"Red flags" of fever, night pain, prolonged morning stiffness, bone pain, or cramps identify systemic illnesses that are causing back pain.**

- **Your lumbar spine has 5 vertebrae (L1– L5) and discs supported by ligaments and muscles.**

- **Your spinal cord is the communications center for transmitting pain impulses and messages between your body and brain.**

- **Pain travels: injury in one structure, such as a joint, can cause pain in another structure, such as a muscle connected on the same nerve network.**

- **Your perception of pain can vary for many reasons, including your level of stress.**

- **When your back is weak you are at more risk for injury. The major muscle supporting your lower back is among the weakest in your body.**

Dr. B—

2

WORKING WITH YOUR DOCTOR

Your doctor needs a complete picture of you and your back pain before he or she can get to the bottom of the problem. During the telling of your story and a physical examination, any one fact may be the clue that solves the puzzle of your back pain. In fact, most diagnoses are established during the history portion of the examination. The rest of the process identifies the correct diagnosis from the variety of possibilities developed by your description of your back pain.

Your age and gender, naturally, are important to a correct diagnosis. For example, more herniated discs occur between the ages of twenty-five and forty-five. Conversely, approximately 80 percent of people with cancer of the spine are fifty or older. Men have back pain more frequently than women, some of which may be explained by occupational exposure to more physically strenuous work. Certain disorders occur exclusively or predominantly in women, such as back pain during pregnancy and osteoporosis. (Men are at risk for this thinning of the bones, too, but the risk is greater for post-menopausal women.)

The history you provide is the most important part of the diagnostic process. The more complete the information, the greater its value. Every subsequent step is used to confirm the ideas and even hunches developed during the medical history. The first part of your history, the chief complaint, is your description of what brought you to the doctor. In most circumstances, the chief complaint is "I have a pain in my back." Another frequent chief complaint is "I have a pain in my back that runs down my leg to my foot." Your description guides the doctor's questions.

Telling your story allows you to describe those events that you believe are most important in explaining the evolution of your back pain. Your doctor may or may not ask questions as you progress with your narrative. A physician may interrupt to ask a question if a particular point is essential to differentiate between diagnostic possibilities. For example, you may be asked: "Did the pain that ran down your leg go to your big toe or small toe?"

Help yourself and your doctor by gathering your thoughts about your back pain and organizing the description of your symptoms and questions you want to ask. Perhaps you can store the information in your head, but writing it down may be more useful. By carefully thinking about your back pain, you will have organized information necessary to start the diagnostic process. Also, bring a list of your medicines—or the actual medicines—with you and the names and addresses of your other healthcare providers.

QUESTIONS TO HELP YOU FIND THE CAUSE

When Did the Pain Begin?

Acute onset of back pain is most closely associated with a specific episode of trauma to the spine, such as lifting a heavy bag of groceries from the back seat of your car. In contrast, systemic illnesses cause pain that is gradual in onset. People with inflammatory arthritis of the spine (spondyloarthropathy) may have had back stiffness and pain for six months or longer when first evaluated for their spine symptoms.

How Long Does It Last and How Often Does It Occur?

The initial episodes of mechanical low back pain resolve over days. With successive episodes, the duration of pain increases to a week and then a month; episodes may be intermittent over time. The frequency of pain follows environmental exposure, such as shoveling snow in winter or several hours of weeding the garden in the summer.

For medical low back pain, the important characteristic is duration, not frequency. As opposed to the short duration of mechanical low back pain, medical low back pain is more persistent. It may last for months, with minimal variation in discomfort.

Where Is It Located and Where Else Do You Feel It?

Most low back pain is localized between the lower rib and buttocks, where the spinal curve (lordosis) is greatest. Frequently, the pain starts to one side of the spine and quickly spreads across the low back. The fleshy part of the back is more commonly affected than the bones themselves. Occasionally pain will be present on both sides of the spine, near the "dimples" just above the buttocks, over the sacroiliac joints. Sometimes the location and radiation of pain is very difficult to describe because it is referred pain, that is, it comes from somewhere else (see chapter 1). Pain can move side to side, or up and down the leg. However, the most important facts are where the pain first started and how far the pain has spread.

What Makes It Feel Worse or Better?

Mechanical low back pain disorders improve with rest and worsen with certain activities. Muscle injuries are aggravated with stretching and are relieved when the muscle is at rest and therefore shortened in length. This resting position allows healing to take place. For example, a thirty-two-year-old man who picked up a heavy box of papers experienced immediate onset of right-sided low back pain. His pain increased with any movement of his spine forward (flexed) or to the left side. These motions stretched the injured muscles on the right side of his spine, thereby intensifying the pain. He was most comfortable when resting in bed or standing with a tilt to the right side.

Anything that increases pressure on discs will also increase compression of spinal nerves. If you have a herniated disc, you have increased pain with sitting, sneezing, coughing, or having a bowel movement. Disc pressure is reduced when you are standing up.

If you have more back pain standing, then you could have arthritis of the back joints. You probably have less pain when you sit. When leg pain occurs with standing, spinal stenosis is the most common diagnosis. Walking for a distance may be associated with leg pain. If you sit down or rest against a structure with your spine bent forward, your leg pain decreases.

Alleviating and aggravating factors for medical low back pain are more complicated. Inflammatory arthritis can hurt more when you are not moving and hurt less with walking, bending, and stretching. Others with medical low back pain have severe low back pain unless they stay motionless. They may also have other signs of a serious illness such as fever, chills, or weight loss (remember those red flags).

What Time of Day or Night Does It Occur?

Systemic disorders, like inflammatory arthritis, are most symptomatic during sleep or in the early morning while getting out of bed. Stiffness and pain are improved with normal movement as the day progresses. Conversely, people with tumors of the spine have increased pain when lying flat in bed. They usually sit in a chair to sleep, or they may walk around to relieve their pain.

Mechanical disorders become more symptomatic with use, and the greatest pain occurs at the end of the day.

What Is the Quality and Intensity?

A wide variety of terms are used to describe pain. Skin disorders cause local burning pain on the surface of the body. Disorders of the bones, joints, muscles, and ligaments cause a deep, dull ache that is most intense over the involved site. A cramping pain is associated with reflex contraction of an injured muscle, or from a muscle chronically contracted to protect an injured portion of the lumbar spine, like a facet joint.

Pain from nerve compression (radicular pain) has a sharp, shooting, burning quality that follows the distribution of the compressed nerve. This kind of pain is associated with sciatica, compression of the sciatic nerve. Other forms of nerve pain occur with direct trauma to the nerve or secondary to changes in the metabolism of the nerve, a situation associated with diabetes. This form of pain has a tingling and crushing component that is unaffected by physical position of the body but is intensified by touching of the skin supplied by the nerve. The severity of the pain may continue even after the stimulus is gone.

Kidney stones cause a recurrent gripping pain that rises quickly to its greatest intensity in twenty to thirty seconds, lasts one to two minutes, and then quickly resolves. Throbbing pain is associated with disorders of blood vessels. A tearing sensation is a potential sign of blood vessel injury that may cause loss of blood flow to structures in the lower extremities.

Who Else in Your Family Has It?

Most disorders of the lumbar spine are not genetic. However, disc herniations and sciatica occurring in many family members suggests a relationship between your back and leg pain and family characteristics. The group of conditions known as inflammatory arthritis of the spine (spondyloarthropathies) has a genetic predisposition and a test could determine if you are at risk. Therefore, mention these disorders to your doctor as part of your family history.

How Does Your Work or Lifestyle Affect It?

Your profession can determine your risk for developing low back pain. Other risk factors aside, heavy lifting and carrying on the job add to the risk for developing mechanical low back pain. Onset of pain while at work has potential implications for qualifying for worker's compensation. Be sure to tell your doctor if you see a relationship between your job and your back pain. If you sit all day at a computer, you may develop low back pain, and there's been lots of talk lately about ergonomics, posture chairs, and mouse pads. (See my Back School FAQ for information about chairs.)

Smoking tobacco and drinking alcohol are implicated in osteoporosis; they weaken the bones in your spine. (Alcohol may also limit the use of certain medications used to control pain and inflammation.) Think about the way your back pain affects activities and relationships with the important people in your life. Perhaps you are unable to participate in your basketball or bowling league or swing dancing. Back pain often has a detrimental effect on sexual relationships. When any simple motion increases your pain it is difficult to enjoy sex. Discuss these social and personal difficulties honestly with your physician, so he or she can help you.

Past and Present Medical History

Your medical history necessarily deals with past and current illnesses. For example, a history of cancer may have great significance in the onset of new back pain. A previous injury, such as slipping and falling on ice, may be the initiating event in the development of a herniated disc. A history of diabetes increases risk for developing nerve irritation (neuropathy) that causes back and leg pain. Psoriasis and inflammatory bowel disease are associated with inflammatory arthritis of the spine. Eye inflammation may also be linked with back disorders. Illnesses such as hypertension may limit the use of certain medications because of side effects. Environmental or drug allergies should be mentioned as well.

THE PHYSICAL EXAMINATION

Once your pain story and medical and family histories have been obtained, you will move on to the second part of the diagnostic process—the physical examination of your lower back. Physicians each have their own methods for this examination, but here's what I look for.

SCOLIOSIS

Lumbar Spine Examination

Your doctor will examine your spine while you are standing, sitting, and lying on your stomach to discover any abnormalities. Curvature of the spine (scoliosis) is associated with elevation of either shoulder and is best discovered when standing (fig. 2.1). Tilting the pelvis will show inequality in the length of the legs. From the side, it is easy to note a forward position of the head with a mound at attachment of the neck to the chest, which is known as a dowager's hump, or increased backward curve of the spine, *kyphosis* (fig. 2.2). Characteristics of poor posture are also best seen from the side. For example, if you have a protruding abdomen, it's a sign of weak abdominal muscles and you will have an increased lumbar curve, or hyperlordosis.

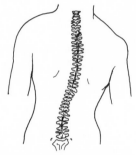

Figure 2.1 Scoliosis has curved this spine to the right in the thoracic region and to the left in the low back. Notice the left shoulder is higher than the right shoulder. When bending forward, the left shoulder blade will be more prominent than the right. This structural abnormality affects young girls and is most effectively treated when identified early.

Your doctor will touch your back with varying degrees of pressure to detect increased muscle contraction or spasm. Back muscles at rest can be compressed with gentle pressure because they are soft and moveable. Muscles in spasm are tense and firm to the touch and may be tender with direct palpation. More commonly, moving the tense muscle increases pain.

Both sides of your spine will be compressed to examine for symmetry of muscle contraction. In the resting upright position, spasm on one side of the lumbar spine may be detected while the other side of the spine is normal. This asymmetry of muscle contraction helps identify the location of the original injury, most often to muscle or fascia.

KYPHOSIS

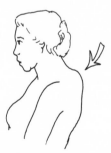

Figure 2.2 Kyphosis, a prominent bump between the shoulder blades, pushes the head forward.

Range of Motion and Rhythm

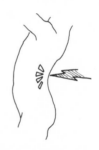

Tests for range of motion can tell us a great deal. For example, if you have increased back pain when you bend backward you may have arthritis of the facet joints (fig. 2.3). Thigh pain may also be an indication of abnormalities in organs located in the back of the abdomen. You

Figure 2.3 Bending the lumbar spine backward is called extension.

will be asked to bend forward from a standing position, bend to both sides, bend backward, and rotate your hips. (The total range of motion of the spine is not always as important as the natural rhythm of motion.)

An injured lumbar spine will have limited normal motion because the muscles will tighten to protect it. The lumbar spine will not have the normal curve in the standing position, nor will the lumbar curve reverse. Forward movement of the spine is severely limited. If injury to the spine is unilateral, the spine is tilted to the side of the shortened muscles in spasm. There may also be limited ability to bend the knees (flexion), which results from tightness of the buttocks and hamstring muscles in the back of the thigh.

When you bend and return to an upright position, the motion can reveal information about the injured structures causing pain. Normally, the hips are rotated first, and the lower spine goes from being bent forward to bent backward. When an injury affects the spine, the spine is bent backward first, and bending the knees and rotating the hips establish the upright posture (fig. 2.4).

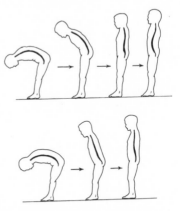

Bending to one side stretches the muscles on the opposite side of your spine and compresses spinal joints on the same side as the motion. Pain just to the side of the midline on the same side as the motion suggests irritation of the facet joint at that level of the spine. Pain from

Figure 2.4 Normally, bending backward and simultaneously rotating your hips (upper panel) is a fluid and effortless motion. When your back is in pain, however, the motion is abnormal (lower panel) and relies on rotating your hips and bending your knees. This motion is hesitant and fatiguing.

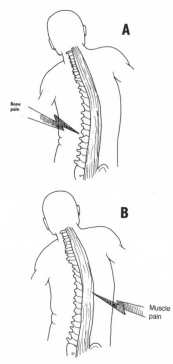

Figure 2.5 When pain is on the same side (A) as the direction of movement, it is associated with bone pain from facet joint disease. Pain on the opposite side as the direction of movement (B) is associated with a muscle injury.

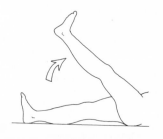

Figure 2.6 By raising your leg straight, you stretch the sciatic nerve. In this position, pain that radiates below your knee may indicate a herniated disc.

compression of the facet joint may radiate down the leg to the foot. A stretching sensation with pain on the side opposite the motion suggests a muscle injury with spasm (fig. 2.5).

Testing Muscles and Reflexes

When you are lying flat on your back on the examining table, your doctor may raise your leg up in the air. This maneuver puts a strain on your sciatic nerve (fig. 2.6), so if there is nerve compression, your leg pain will get worse with this test. If the pain is not in your leg, but in your lower back or buttock, this suggests a problem in joints or muscles without nerve irritation. The doctor may bend your knee and rotate your leg from side to side while you lie on your side. This movement tests the integrity of your hip, and arthritis in the hip causes pain in the groin and buttock.

The sensory and reflex examination is done while you are seated with your legs dangling. The doctor will touch both your legs with a pin or a tuning fork and ask if you can tell the difference in sensation. This helps pinpoint which nerve is causing numbness. Numbness between the legs is associated with disorders of the lower sacral nerve roots. Hitting your knee and the back of your ankle with a rubber hammer is another test of reflexes. An absence of knee reflex, for example, corresponds to an abnormality of the L-4 nerve root.

Toe raises repeated ten times determine a difference in strength in the calf muscles. Walking on your heels tests the stamina of your shin muscles and big toe. A deep knee bend tests the strength of all your lower extremity muscles (fig. 2.7).

Other Tests

A targeted musculoskeletal examination will concentrate on the lumbar spine and may not evaluate other portions of the skeletal system. However, if you have joint pain in other areas, then it is appropriate to examine all the joints.

In addition to the joints, other organ systems may be evaluated if the medical history has identified specific disorders such as heart failure or gastrointestinal ulcers. A rectal examination may be necessary if loss of bowel control has occurred along with back pain. This examination is also appropriate for determining the status of the prostate gland in a man with persistent back pain.

The history and physical examination are often all we need to determine the likely cause of a back attack and additional tests are unnecessary before starting therapy. However, X ray and blood tests potentially corroborate the initial impression gained through the medical evaluation. (The next chapter outlines what these tests can and cannot do.)

DOCTORS AND HEALTH CARE PROFESSIONALS WHO TREAT LOW BACK PAIN

I am a rheumatologist. Rheumatology is a subspecialty of internal medicinedealing with the treatment of patients with arthritis or any disorders in the bones, joints, or muscles. We prescribe nonsteroidal anti-inflammatory drugs (NSAIDs—aspirin-like drugs), muscle relaxants, and physical therapy. To find a rheumatologist in your community, either an M.D. or D.O., check with your local Arthritis Foundation or the American College of Rheumatology.

A number of other physicians and health care professionals take care of back pain patients.

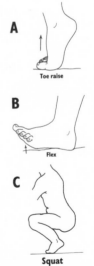

Figure 2.7 These three tests measure the strength of the calf (A), shin (B), and thigh (C).

- Internist/Family practitioner: An allopathic (M.D.) or osteopathic (D.O.) physician who is a primary care professional offering general health care needs, including general back therapy.

- Neurologist: M.D. or D.O. specializing in the diagnosis and treatment of nerve disorders; this doctor has special skills in the diagnosis of nerve abnormalities, including electrodiagnostic tests.

- Physiatrist: M.D. or D.O. specializing in rehabilitation of the musculoskeletal and nervous systems, who offers special skills in electrodiagnostic tests, exercise methods, and body supports.

- Orthopedic surgeon: M.D. or D.O. who is a specialist in the surgery of the skeletal system, including the spine

- Neurosurgeon: M.D. or D.O. specializing in the surgery of the nervous system, including the spine.

- Physical Therapist: P.T., R.P.T. (Registered), or M.P.T. (Masters) specializing in the use of exercise and physical methods to relieve pain and restore function

- Chiropractor: D.C. (Doctor of Chiropractic) who uses physical adjustments and mobilization to treat spinal disorders.

- Acupuncturist: A health professional who places needles at various points of the body to unblock energy to treat spinal disorders.

- Massage therapist: L.M.T. (Licensed massage therapist) who uses therapeutic muscle massage to improve musculoskeletal disorders.

Chose your health care provider depending on your specific back problem, but always start with your primary care physician or rheumatologist. See a surgeon if you have muscle weakness or have failed medical therapy.

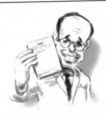

DR. B'S PRESCRIPTION SUMMARY

R

- The most important part of the back evaluation is your own complete medical and lifestyle history

- The specific character of back pain helps define its source.

- The physical examination identifies abnormalities of normal movement, sensation, muscle strength, and reflexes.

- Most back evaluations do not require additional X ray or blood tests.

- Your primary care physician or rheumatologist can start your back evaluation and offer appropriate referrals if additional therapy is needed.

Dr. B—

3

WHAT DIAGNOSTIC TESTS CAN—AND CANNOT—TELL YOU

When new patients come to my office, I always pick up their charts from the plastic holder on the door to the examining room. This plastic holder may also contain a large envelope of X rays or magnetic resonance imaging (MRI) studies of the lumbar spine. I peruse the chart to familiarize myself with the patient I'm about to meet, but I do not open the large folder and study the test results.

After introducing myself, I ask new patients to tell me the reason they scheduled an appointment. They usually respond by mentioning their back pain, then they ask if I have reviewed the X rays and MRI results they brought. Invariably, I see their disappointment when I tell them I have not looked at these tests. This disappointment is understandable, because they have gone to the trouble of supplying the information and believe they are being "good patients." However, there is a method to what may seem like madness. Patients eventually understand my thinking when I explain why I like to hear about their problems and examine them first before reviewing their X rays or MRI results.

Diagnostic "pictures" have importance only in the context of your current clinical complaints. Any number of abnormalities may appear on the X rays or MRI, but these results may be of little consequence in explaining and treating the problem that prompted a visit to a new doctor.

I repeat this scenario with patients again and again, and it serves to shed light on both the advantages and disadvantages of rapid advancements in medical technology. We now have the ability to look inside the human body and obtain highly detailed images without exposing people to radiation. The MRI scanner uses large magnets and radio waves and presents visual images of the structures in the spine that were difficult to see with older, radiation-based technology. The computed axial tomography scan (CT) uses X rays (radiation) to identify structures in and around the spine. We can put multiple CT pictures together to achieve a three-dimensional view of the spine.

Pictures May Not Tell the Whole Story

Most of us are impressed by what these imaging machines can do, and no question, they represent important progress in medicine. But just because we can see the spine in better ways than ever before does not mean that we have significantly increased our understanding of what causes back pain.

Our enthusiasm for medical technology must be tempered by recognizing that changes or deviations from what we define as "normal" are not necessarily associated with a specific complaint. In fact, most changes from normal are asymptomatic. Patients may tell me that an MRI scan has documented bulging discs at two or three levels. They are concerned that their bulging discs must be the source of their pain. However, a number of X ray studies have discovered bulging discs at multiple levels of the spine in people *without* any back pain.

The lack of correlation between clinical symptoms and X ray findings is characteristic of the most common causes of low back pain, which are mechanical disorders of the lumbar spine. Based on autopsy findings, by age fifty up to 95 percent of adults show evidence of changes in the spine due to aging, including disc space narrowing. In X ray studies of people fifty or older, 87 percent have demonstrated changes in the intervertebral discs, due again, to aging.

In 1984, the medical journal *Spine* reported research findings that remain important in our understanding that the reason for pain may not be related to what we can see on a picture. This study compared X ray test results of 238 patients with back pain and 66 without pain. In terms of the prevalence of disc degeneration, researchers could detect no difference between the two groups.

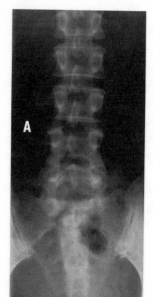

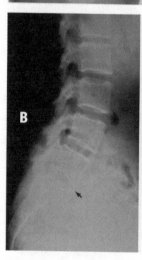

Figure 3.1 From the front, this plain X-ray of a lumbar spine (A) reveals no abnormalities. From the side, however (B), we can see a mild narrowing of the last vertebral body and the sacrum (black arrow). This narrowing indicates disc degeneration.

Always keep in mind that many changes in the spine that are detectable through X ray testing do not cause pain, while other abnormalities have significant consequences and require further evaluation. What remains important is knowing when to get X ray testing and what such testing says about the health of the spine. Most people with back pain get better without any of these tests.

CONVENTIONAL X RAYS

Generally, you will not require X rays of the lumbar spine during the early stages of your back attack except when there are signs of a medical cause of back pain. These are the red flags mentioned earlier and include fever, weight loss, or history of cancer. In most circumstances, X rays are not required unless you've been in pain for six to eight weeks.

I order X rays of the lumbar spine if I am concerned about medical disorders of the spine, including arthritis that affects the facet joints. I do not order X rays if a soft tissue problem such as muscle strain is causing pain. If pain has been present for more than four to six weeks, or for individuals over age fifty with persistent pain, then X ray testing is usually called for.

Generally, you will be positioned on your back and on your side for an initial X ray study. Oblique (on an incline) views, required less frequently, are taken with the X ray tube at a forty-five-degree slant to your body. If there is a concern about the stability of your spine, you may have flexion (bending forward) and extension (bending backward) views of the lumbar spine. In your day-to-day activities, these bending motions place forces on the spine that may cause shifting of the vertebrae if they are not fully anchored by the facet joints (spondylolisthesis). A routine view of the pelvis, which images the sacroiliac and hip joints, is taken while you are flat on the X ray table.

Plain X rays are excellent at photographing the spatial arrangement of the vertebrae (fig. 3.1), and they show the distance between vertebrae, which indicates the health of the corresponding disc. These pictures also detect changes in bony architecture that may be altered by the presence of prostate or breast cancer or osteoporosis.

Modern X ray testing equipment does the same work as older machinery but minimizes exposure to radiation while remaining the least expensive radiographic technique. The cost of lumbar spine series ranges from $180 to $300.

MAGNETIC RESONANCE IMAGING (MRI)

MRI is the most recently developed diagnostic imaging technique for medical conditions such as low back pain. Through the use of radio waves and magnets, with some strengths greater than the magnetic field around the Earth, this non-invasive technique images the component parts of the lumbar spine from a number of directions. The anatomy of the intervertebral disc, spinal nerves, ligaments, facet joints, and adjacent muscles are visualized (fig. 3.2), and intervertebral disc herniations are easily identified.

Contrast dye (gadolinium) may be injected into a vein if additional information is needed to determine the amount of blood flow to a specific area of the spine. Increased blood flow occurs in areas where scarring from previous back surgeries or tumors is present.

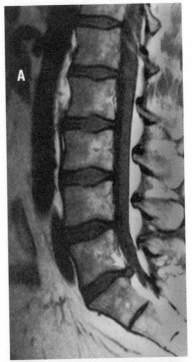

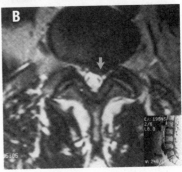

Figure 3.2 With an MRI view from the side of this lumbar spine (A) we can see that there is a disc herniation at the L5-S interspace (white arrow). A cross-sectional view (B) identifies the disc herniation on the left side (white arrow).

You are on your back during an MRI and placed in a confining, hollow tube. Depending on the number of views needed, the test lasts between twenty and sixty minutes, and the machine makes a ticking sound during the scans.

For those with claustrophobia, an open MRI is available, but the images are less sharp than those produced by the closed "tube" version.

The MRI is a painless procedure, but if you are experiencing back pain you may be uncomfortable lying still on your back with your legs straight for the length of time needed to complete the examination. MRI involves no exposure to radiation, but it is not used if you have metal clips with magnetic properties in your body from surgery. There is a risk that the clips will move under the influence of the magnet. The MRI machine will also short-circuit a pacemaker.

The cost of an MRI ranges from approximately $1,300 to $2,600, and the higher figure is associated with the cost of two MRIs, one with and one without contrast. MRI scanners are available in most communities with a local hospital.

I can offer a personal perspective on this test because I had one myself. The top of the tube was about two inches from my face, which is why those with claustrophobia have a difficult time with this test. I was told to remain still while the scans were completed. I frequently gazed toward my feet to assure myself that escape from the machine was possible. I was very glad to get out of the tube once the scans were over. Because of this experience, I am able to sympathize with my back pain patients who must undergo this test while they experience back discomfort. I promised myself that I would not send my patients for MRI testing unless the information was essential to their care.

MRIs are appropriate for those who have red flags for medical disorders and for those with sciatica (pain radiating from the back to the leg) who are considering epidural corticosteroid injections (see chapter 7) or lumbar spine surgery (see chapter 10). Bone abnormalities are better visualized by another radiographic technique.

The MRI scan is the most sensitive test for those who need radiographic evaluation to identify the location of the disc herniation and nerve compression. X rays may be entirely normal in individuals with a herniated disc, but MRI scans identify the location of disc herniations including the migration of extruded disc fragments. A CT scan can identify disc herniations in individuals who have metal in their bodies and are therefore unable to undergo MRI testing, but the CT does not offer the general overview of the spine that is obtained with the MRI machine.

COMPUTED AXIAL TOMOGRAPHY (CT)

CT scans, sometimes called CAT scans, create cross-sectional (axial) images of the bony structure of the lumbar spine (fig. 3.3). With a computer, the images can be reformatted to form a three-dimensional model of the spine. CT scans also assess soft tissues including discs, ligaments, nerve roots, and fat. CT technology is appropriate for people with pacemakers, metal clips, or claustrophobia, who are therefore unable to have an MRI scan.

CT scans are taken while you lie flat on your back in the center of an open circular overhead structure that supports the scanning machine (gantry). This test does not cause pain except for the discomfort of lying still for twenty to forty minutes. Radiation exposure is three to five rads, with the greater exposure associated with higher-resolution scans. The cost ranges from $800 to $2,000, if a myelogram is required.

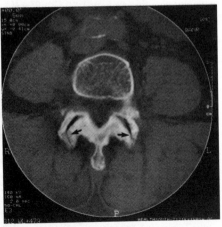

Figure 3.3 A cross-sectional view with a CT scan reveals arthritis in both facet joints (arrows).

CT findings corroborate clinical impressions, but as with MRI results, abnormalities not associated with symptoms may be present in as many as 30 percent of people without pain. I order CT scans to reveal bony abnormalities occurring with central and lateral spinal stenosis (compression of spinal nerves), facet joint arthritis, fractures, and metastatic bone disease. CT is my second choice of image testing for identifying a herniated disc and by necessity is the first option for those with a pacemaker or claustrophobia.

MYELOGRAPHY

Before the advent of MRI technology, the myelogram was the "gold standard" for X ray evaluation of the lumbar spine. The myelogram fell out of favor for a number of reasons, one of which is the need to inject a contrast dye into the spinal canal, thereby making it an invasive test. A headache may develop after the exam and in rare circumstances a seizure can be caused by the dye. Despite its limitations, the myelogram allows you to stand or bend while the films are exposed. The ability to test in a "functional" position is particularly helpful for diagnosing spinal stenosis. Myelography is also an important radiographic technique for spinal surgery patients with metal rods because the presence of metal spoils the ability of MRI or CT scans to visualize the spine.

Like MRI and CT, myelography is associated with anatomical abnormalities without pain. Just like the other tests, clinical judgement is important in evaluating the myelogram. I rarely order a myelogram or CT-myelogram and only use the test for patients considering surgery for spinal stenosis and who want to know the extent of the bone removal required to improve their condition.

Because the dye eventually becomes diluted, a myelogram must be completed in twenty to thirty minutes. However, because of the spinal puncture, you must sit for two hours and then lie down for two hours. Resting in these positions diminishes the risk of headaches. X ray exposure is six to seven rads, and the cost is approximately $1,200.

BONE SCAN

Bone scan (radionuclide imaging) is a useful test to detect bone abnormalities or fractures. The bone scan involves an injection of a small amount of a radioactive material into your vein. A few hours following the injection, the scanning portion of the test begins. You are flat on your stomach for up to sixty minutes while the lumbar spine is scanned. Areas of the skeleton that are reacting to an injury (fracture or inflammation) show up as a dark or "hot" spot on the scan. Most bone cells in the skeleton are in a dormant state maintaining bone structure. The increased activity on the scan results from the increased absorption of the radioactive material by the bone cells trying to heal the injury. The presence of the "hot" spot does not indicate a specific diagnosis, because tumors, infections, fractures, and arthritis all cause dark spots on the scans. Additional radiographic evaluation or blood testing is needed to reach a specific diagnosis.

I order bone scans when I am concerned about the possibility of bone fractures in the spine. Some fractures are very small and are not seen by plain X rays. Bone scans are able to identify the location of these fractures regardless of the cause.

A bone scan is painless except for the discomfort associated with being flat for a period of time, which may increase your back pain. The radiation exposure is small, 0.15 rad, and the cost is approximately $600.

DISCOGRAPHY

I do not recommend discography, but if you are thinking about surgery, you may be asked by the surgeon to undergo this test. Before you do, ask the doctor what information will be gained from the test and what effect it will have on your surgery.

Discography may identify the specific disc level causing pain. It is both a radiographic and therapeutic technique performed by placing a thin needle into a disc, followed by the injection of dye first and anesthetic medication second. The amount of dye required to fill the space, the appearance of the dye in the disc, and reproduction of your back pain are important pieces of information generated by this test. If your back pain is generated by the first injection, a second injection with anesthetic is given in an attempt to relieve your discomfort. Pain relief from medication is also characteristic of a positive test. The test is used to determine the source of back pain when other radiographic techniques have not produced conclusive results.

The procedure is done using a fluoroscope to determine the placement of the needle as it is moved into the disc. The length of the procedure depends on the number of discs studied. Radiation exposure is two rads; the cost is approximately $600.

BONE DENSITOMETRY

This is a useful way to measure bone mass; low bone mass resulting from a loss of calcium from the bone is associated with increased risk for fracture. Dual X ray absorptiometry (DXA) is the method most frequently used to determine bone mineral density in the spine and the thigh bone. Low-energy X rays are used to determine the difference in the absorption of the beam by the bone versus the soft tissues. Bone tissue will absorb the beam of X rays, whereas X rays will pass through the soft tissues. The difference in absorption corresponds to the amount of calcium in the bones. The best candidates for this test are postmenopausal women, and men and women taking corticosteroids.

You will be flat on your back on a table during this test while the arm of the machine passes over you for about twenty to thirty minutes. This test measures both the lumbar spine and hip. The amount of radiation is low, 0.1 rad, and the cost is approximately $280.

ELECTRODIAGNOSTIC TESTS

Electrodiagnostic tests are useful to confirm the suspicion of nerve compression and are commonly used to evaluate peripheral nerves that travel beyond the spinal cord. These tests are also used to detect muscle and nerve damage; they demonstrate abnormalities in nerve and muscle function but do not identify the specific cause of the dysfunction. Electromyogram (EMG) tests evaluate the electrical activity generated by muscles at rest and at work. Nerve conduction velocity (NCV) studies measure the speed of the transmission of the electrical signal in a nerve. Both of these tests are useful in differentiating among the neurologic disorders associated with back and leg pain. These tests are most often needed to evaluate pain that radiates down the leg (radiculopathy).

EMG involves inserting needles into muscles that are supplied by the damaged nerve, as well as other muscles in the back and leg. The process of inserting the needles is painful and requires contracting the muscle after insertion. The amount of irritation and the amount of electricity generated by the muscle help determine the degree of injury to the nerve.

Damage does not occur as soon as the nerve is injured, and abnormalities may take a week or more to appear. For example, disc compression on a nerve may take days before the muscle supplied by that nerve has abnormal electrical signals. Therefore, electrodiagnostic tests done too early will miss the abnormality. EMG tests may take two to four weeks before being helpful. Once a nerve is damaged, the number of nerve fibers supplying a muscle diminish even if the nerve compression is removed. That change in nerve function, measured by an EMG, may be permanent. No X ray radiation is associated with an EMG test, but it is associated with pain with the insertion of needles into tested muscles. An EMG procedure takes about sixty minutes to complete. The cost ranges from $32 to $376, depending on the number of muscles tested.

NCV studies determine the speed of the signal as it travels through the nerves in the legs or arms. Surface electrodes that look like felt pads are placed over a muscle in the foot. Another pad is placed over the same nerve in a location further up the leg. These pads can be moved over different locations on the limb where the nerve can be pinched by structures in the leg. An electrical signal is generated in the pad closer to the center of the body. The signal is detected at the distal pad and the speed of conduction is matched against normal velocities. Slowing of the speed with which the signal is transferred down the leg determines areas of compression of the nerve outside of the spinal canal. The cost of this test ranges from $58 to $580, depending on the number of nerve conductions tested.

While electrodiagnostic tests document the presence of nerve dysfunction, they do not determine the specific cause. An abnormal EMG documents the location of nerve damage and helps the surgeon identify individuals for whom surgery is likely to bring improvement. NCV differentiates between spinal cord problems and peripheral nerve disorders. I order these tests when I need to determine the exact level of nerve dysfunction in order to provide guidance to anesthesiologists for therapeutic injections or to surgeons for the area of spine surgery.

BLOOD TESTS

Since most of my patients have mechanical low back pain, which does not cause abnormalities detected in blood tests, these laboratory tests are seldom needed. However, they are necessary when red flags are identified. Only a few blood tests are useful for identifying abnormalities associated with medical back pain. These include: an erythrocyte sedimentation rate (ESR), C-reactive protein (CRP), complete blood count (CBC), and blood chemistries.

ESR is a simple test that measures the speed that red blood cells fall in a tube. Centuries ago, Hippocrates, the Greek physician whom we call the "father of medicine," commented that blood that separated and settled into a clear part and a red part was associated with an ill person. Red blood cells fall because they are coated with an increased level of proteins that are generated because of inflammation anywhere in the body. The inflammation may indicate infection, a tumor, or inflammatory arthritis, which are not mechanical disorders. The normal ESR level is less than 10 mm/hour in men and 20 mm/hour in women. ESR greater than 100 mm/hour is often associated with tumors. ESR may return toward normal as the underlying disorder is treated and improves.

CRP is a protein produced by the liver when inflammation is present, and CRP may rise before the ESR becomes elevated. The normal level of CRP is less than 0.2 mg/100 ml. Levels between 1 and 10 mg/100 ml are moderate increases; levels over 10 are markedly elevated. Levels of CRP remain elevated in chronic inflammatory states. Elevated ESR or CRP call for more intense evaluation in order to determine the medical cause of low back pain.

CBC (red and white blood cells and platelets) and chemistry tests are more often performed to monitor toxicity of drugs than to identify the cause of back pain. Nonsteroidal anti-inflammatory drugs often are prescribed to treat low back pain, and those who take these drugs for an extended period of time are given blood tests to monitor the hematocrit and liver and kidney function.

Medical history, physical examination, and X ray and blood tests allow your doctor to separate mechanical and medical causes of low back pain and set you on the road to recovery—whether with basic care you can provide yourself, or with further medical treatment.

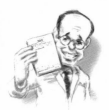

DR. B'S PRESCRIPTION SUMMARY

R

- Plain X rays reveal a specific diagnosis in only a small number of back pain sufferers.

- MRI is the best technique to identify soft tissue abnormalities in nerves, bone marrow, and muscles.

- CT scan is the best technique for showing bone abnormalities.

- Bone scan is the best survey technique to evaluate the entire skeleton for abnormal bone activity.

- Electrodiagnostic tests identify the location of nerve damage.

- Blood tests help distinguish mechanical from medical low back pain.

Dr. B—

PART TWO:
KNOWING YOUR TREATMENT OPTIONS

4

THE BASIC BACK PAIN RELIEF PROGRAM

My basic therapy for low back and leg pain can work for you as long as your pain is not from a systemic illness. Pain from a mechanical disorder such as muscle strain, joint irritation, herniated disc, or hip arthritis, for example, can improve if you control physical activities, use over-the-counter pain medications, stay fit with aerobic exercise, and—most importantly—self-educate. If your back pain improves, you probably won't need any more evaluation to speed your recovery. If you are in doubt about your recovery, contact your physician immediately.

CONTROL PHYSICAL ACTIVITIES BUT LIMIT BED REST

In the past we were told to lie down if we had back pain, to let the muscles rest and heal. This is wrong! Now we know that bed rest is no better to resolve back pain than being up and walking around. Movement seems to help the tissues of the back heal more rapidly, too. Extended bed rest, on the other hand, deconditions the heart, lungs, stomach, and skeletal muscles. So keep bed rest to a minimum. Studies have shown that two days of bed rest is as good as seven days of bed rest for the relief of back pain. The benefits of bed rest are also limited if pain travels to your leg. In a study of 183 people with sciatica from a herniated disc, people given bed rest for two weeks did no better than those allowed to walk around.

On the other hand, being out of bed does not mean returning to your usual daily work and recreational activities. Stay home from work until you are able to walk or stand for thirty minutes without pain, and you feel comfortable sitting for twenty to thirty minutes without increased pain. If you have acute low back pain, limit your activities and you will have a faster recovery and be much less likely to have chronic or recurrent episodes of low back pain. Increase activity as pain decreases.

Bed Rest Positions

When bed rest is indicated, a couple of positions are most comfortable. The semi-Fowler position places the least pressure on spinal discs, joints, and muscles: Put a small pillow behind your head and two to three pillows under your knees to flex your hips and knees. Your mattress should be firm, but it may feel better to lie on a comforter on the floor.

Get Out of Bed Carefully

Another comfortable position is on your side with a flat back, with your legs curled up with a pillow between your knees. This is a side semi-Fowler position and is the way to get into and out of bed. Push against the bed with your lower arm while letting your legs slide off the edge of the bed. The weight of your legs will swing your chest up with the help of your lower arm. To get back into bed, do the reverse. Shift your upper body weight to the palm of your hand resting on the bed. Slowly let your body down, shifting your weight to your forearm, elbow, and shoulder while you swing your legs up to the bed. Keep your back straight.

Don't Sleep on Your Stomach

This position is particularly stressing on the lumbar spine because it increases the curve and tends to stretch the muscles in the pelvis, causing more pain. If you have to sleep on your stomach, put a pillow or two under your abdomen. This will flatten your spine and place less pressure on the psoas muscle in the pelvis.

USING OVER-THE-COUNTER MEDICATIONS

The final goal of all therapies is to achieve a back that is painless and functional without drugs. Once maximum function has been reached, medicines can be gradually decreased so you can function without them. But do take them to reduce pain so you can keep moving.

Acetaminophen (Tylenol) is a pure pain reliever (analgesic) without any anti-inflammatory effect. The maximum dose is six tablets per day (less if you drink alcohol). The long-acting form of acetaminophen (650 mg) lasts six to eight hours. Acetaminophen is easily tolerated and doesn't upset your stomach. However, for many people, the medication is not powerful enough to decrease pain.

Nonsteroidal anti-inflammatory drugs (NSAID) have pain-relieving and anti-inflammatory effects. Aspirin was the first NSAID and is still a very powerful drug in adequate doses. For example, patients with rheumatoid arthritis will ingest sixteen tablets a day in divided doses. At this dose it is analgesic and anti-inflammatory. At lower doses, aspirin is analgesic with less anti-inflammatory effects. The problem with aspirin is that it irritates the stomach and can cause ulcers with bleeding. It can also have bad effects on kidney function. At toxic doses, aspirin can cause dizziness, loss of hearing, and even coma. If you take aspirin at a dose higher that 81 mg (baby aspirin) for any length of time, you should be evaluated by a physician.

A number of newer NSAIDs are available without a prescription.

- Ibuprofen (Advil, Nuprin, Motrin IB)
- Naproxen (Aleve)
- Ketoprofen (Orudis KT)

The dose for each of these NSAIDs is different, so read the label on the box to determine the effective, safe dose. If one NSAID does not work, try another, because one that helps another person may not help you. If you take an NSAID for two weeks without benefit, then you need to see your doctor. Potential side effects of NSAIDs are that they can cause stomach pain and bleeding, elevations in blood pressure, and decreased function of the kidney in a few people. These drugs need monitoring by your doctor if you take them on a continuous basis.

More potent and more effective NSAIDs are available by prescription. These include the new COX-2 inhibitors, which are as effective as the NSAIDs without as many gastrointestinal side effects.

It is important to understand how long your dose of medicine will be effective, what side effects may occur, and how long you need to remain on a medication. For a full explanation of using drugs for pain, see chapter 7.

APPLIED THERAPY

Cold or Heat

Applying cold or heat in the form of ice massage or wet heat, respectively, is a noninvasive way to improve low back pain. Ice massage is used first to decrease swelling and act as an analgesic. Cold decreases the sensitivity of the sensory fibers, blocking the transmission of pain signals. However, cold tends to stiffen muscles and soft tissue. With an acute muscle strain in the lumbar spine, ice massage for the first forty-eight hours is appropriate. Apply an ice pack, ice for about ten minutes and then remove it. Do this a few times a day.

Heat—wet or dry—can improve blood flow and speed healing. Heat can increase muscle flexibility and improve movement. Personal preference tends to drive the decision regarding dry or wet heat. The important point is not to burn your skin. Leave the heat on for ten to fifteen minutes. The maximum safe exposure is thirty minutes. If you have any circulation problems, speak with your doctor about the amount of time your skin should be exposed to temperature extremes.

If my suggestions for cold and heat applications do not seem to be helping, try the opposite temperature. You may feel better with heat early in the course of a back attack. Or you may be one of the people who have greater pain relief with ice massage for chronic low back pain. Some people use both—ice soon after exercise, and heat an hour or two later.

Corsets

Corsets are wide elastic bands with Velcro fasteners. They come in a variety of widths, with or without heat-molded plastic inserts. Some back pain sufferers use corsets for greater stability to the lumbar spine. The rationale is to increase intra-abdominal pressure in order to decrease the stress on the lumbar spine. Corsets do not keep your lumbar spine motionless. They do remind you to use your legs when lifting, which may be the most important effect of wearing a corset. The downside is that use of a corset will make your muscles weak, so persistent use can be counterproductive.

Wear a corset when you are at risk for excessive strain on your spine, such as with heavy lifting or sitting for long periods of time. Take off the corset as soon as you are out of your risky situation. You must be committed to strengthening exercises once you take off your corset to maintain your back muscles.

AEROBICS: EXPANDING YOUR
COMFORT ZONE—GRADUALLY

Aerobic exercises that improve endurance can help back pain as discomfort starts to decrease. How will you know that you are improving? You will notice that you will feel more comfortable for increasing amounts of time out of bed. You will be able to walk longer distances around your house and outside. As you get better, you will be able to sit for longer periods of time without feeling tired.

Choose an exercise program that you will continue over an extended period of time and something that is easily accessible. You may love to swim, but if there's no pool nearby, this program is not realistic. Exercises most helpful for low back pain are walking, swimming, or riding a stationary bicycle. Before your back pain began, you may have been running instead of walking, or swimming timed laps instead of paddling in the pool, or riding a regular bicycle. I am frequently asked, "How much exercise can I do?" The question is best answered with an explanation of the "Comfort Zone."

Exercise makes these muscles more efficient and the clue to successful training is to use muscles without damaging muscle cells. With damage, the muscles must heal for longer periods of time. This is counterproductive. Finding the fine line between stressing your muscles and causing damage can be difficult. I try to guide my patients to find a happy medium with the concept of the "Comfort Zone."

If you have been exercising and have developed low back pain, cut back your exercise to one tenth of what you were doing before the pain started. For example, if you were walking 10 blocks, you would cut back your exercise to one block. You might say that is no exercise at all, but that amount of exercise would be in the "Comfort Zone." You would do the exercise and would feel no additional soreness the next day. That means you are able to do the exercise safely without causing any damage to the stressed muscles.

Then, every other day increase your exercise another block or another minute. As you increase your effort you will gradually move toward the "Margin Zone." In this zone, the muscles stay sore for a longer period of time measured in hours, but less than a single day. At this point, cut back your exercise slightly to the previous level that did not cause increased soreness. Continue training at the lower level of effort until no soreness remains at the end of the exercise. At that point, the "Comfort Zone" of exercise has been expanded. Increases in times or repetitions are slowed at this point so that your training is between the "Comfort Zone" and the "Margin Zone." Over time you will expand your "Comfort Zone" to increasing levels of exercise.

The goal of this slow progression is to get the benefits of exercise without falling into the "Discomfort Zone." This is where discomfort may last for extended periods of time measured in days. Exercises are discontinued entirely until muscle pain from the exercise has resolved. The trouble with being in this zone is determining the amount of exercise that is safe. It may have been at one block or ten blocks. You cannot tell. That is why starting out in the "Comfort Zone" is so important.

This basic concept can work for any form of exercise—the treadmill, the stair climber, or strength machines. Start out with an amount of exercise that is safe. Once you know that you can complete the exercise without increasing your pain, you can quickly increase your exercise without causing a relapse. I have seen many patients improve with this guidance for their exercise. Try these concepts. I know that you will gain the benefits of exercise with much less risk for reinjury.

The Elusive Last 10 Percent of Recovery

After a while, you will have achieved a significant improvement in your condition with a combination of therapies. Your level of improvement may allow your return to work and most of your recreational activities. However, let's say you have a specific activity that you enjoy. This may be hiking five miles, playing three sets of tennis, or running twenty miles per week. Your activity improvement may be 85 or 90 percent of your original state before back pain occurred. This level of improvement may mean that you are able to hike, but only four miles. Your tennis games may be shorter and less frequent. Your running may be 16 miles on the track at the high school. Your function is not as good as it was prior to your episode of back pain—but it is in the "Comfort Zone." Some people who have had this improvement are not satisfied with their function. They search for the final 10 percent of function. They want to be exactly as they were prior to their back episode.

The difficulty is that this final 10 percent can be difficult to achieve. The search for this 10 percent is as successful as the quest for the Holy Grail. I have seen many patients search for that one elusive therapy that will restore them to their original state. They concentrate on what is lost versus what they have regained. They end up disappointed. Their pessimistic attitude makes it more difficult to reach their goal. People who accept their improvement and work from that point have a better chance to reach their goal. Think about it.

MAINTAIN A POSITIVE ATTITUDE

You may not believe it, but just learning about the causes of back pain and the fact that it gets better on its own has a great therapeutic effect. The positive feelings that come from knowing that your problem will be solved heal low back pain. Understanding the cause of your back pain goes a long way in relieving your anxiety concerning the potential threat to your health. The relief of stress plays an important role in the resolution of back pain, whether acute or chronic. Such knowledge is as powerful as manipulation by a chiropractor or exercises supervised by a physical therapist.

In a study conducted in the state of Washington, researchers assigned 321 people who had back pain for seven days or less to an exercise program supervised by physical therapists, to manipulation treatments given by chiropractors, or to an educational booklet about low back pain. In the first month of the study, the people in the exercise and manipulation programs had less pain. However, at one year, no differences could be found concerning days lost from work or the frequency of additional attacks of low back pain among the groups. The cost of the educational booklet was one third of the expense of the exercise and manipulation therapies. Knowledge is an affordable way to treat low back pain. The people informed about their back pain with the educational booklet needed to go to the doctor less frequently than those who received no information.

You can learn about back pain from this book and others, from videotapes and audiotapes on back exercises, and from the Internet. But be careful on the Internet. There's a great deal of *wrong* information there, so know the reputation of the group presenting the information. I have listed a number of Internet sites from well-regarded professional groups in appendix C. These web sites are updated on a regular basis to offer current information.

One of my patients has taught me the power of a positive attitude. She is ill with a multitude of medical problems, any one of which could devastate a negative person. She returns to my office on a regular basis. She is always nicely dressed and has a smile on her face despite chronic pain and disability. I asked her what her secret was. How in the face of all these difficulties, the chronic nature of her illness, the multiple medicines she needs to take to function, does she continue with such a positive attitude? She told me her secret was very simple. Long ago when her problems started to mount up, she made a choice. She said, "I can be better or bitter. I decided to concentrate on the *e* and not the *i*." She is a testimonial to the therapeutic powers of a positive attitude. Be positive and you can be better even in the face of adversity.

IF BACK PAIN IS CHRONIC

The therapy for chronic low back pain is more complicated. The goal of therapy is maximizing function despite some continued pain. Pain may be exacerbated at times, but this is not necessarily indicative of past or present disease-associated damage.

The Basic Back Pain Relief Program

Chronic back pain can be treated with basic therapy for acute low back pain. Other therapies are added to this basic regimen. Tricyclic antidepressants are sometimes used to increase tone in the pain inhibitory pathway. These drugs also help with the depression that accompanies chronic pain.

If you continue to experience pain, try counterirritant therapy such as TENS, massage, or acupuncture. The relaxation response may decrease the stress associated with chronic pain. Therapies that can result in a relaxation response include yoga, biofeedback, and hypnosis. You and your physician need to meet on a regular basis to modify your therapies to obtain the best outcome.

Some of you reading this book might believe curing a problem is better than controlling it. In all honesty, a cure in human biology is very difficult to achieve. Except for bacterial infections, most human diseases are controlled, not cured. This applies to back pain, too. You may have no pain and function normally. You may think you are cured. However, you are at much greater risk for a second episode of back pain within the next year. That suggests that your back problem has not been cured.

The constant monitoring that comes with controlling a medical problem is a better way to deal with low back pain. Control suggests that you will need to continue to exercise in an appropriate manner to maintain the strength of your back. Although it takes more work on your part, controlling your condition will make you ready to remedy any hint of back pain as soon as it appears.

Despite the best efforts of the human body to heal, many of you will not be better at two, three, or four weeks after the start of an attack of low back pain. Your pain has persisted in the area of the low back, with radiation no farther than the buttock or back of the upper leg. In those circumstances, a visit to a physician is important for an evaluation and additional therapy. As opposed to other health care professionals, a physician is the appropriate practitioner to go to for evaluation and therapy first. Physicians have access to all the diagnostic tools to determine what is wrong with your back. They also have the ability to prescribe all the conventional and complementary therapies that can help acute low back pain. You can read about all of these therapies in the following chapters.

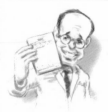

DR. B'S PRESCRIPTION SUMMARY

- Rest in bed only if you have leg pain. Otherwise, limit bed rest and walk as much as you can tolerate.

- Try over-the-counter analgesics and nonsteroidal anti-inflammatory drugs (NSAIDs).

- As your back pain begins to resolve, do low-impact aerobic exercise such as walking or swimming.

- Do not exercise your back too soon after the beginning of a back pain episode. Certain back exercises can increase pain if you do them too early in the healing process. Expand your "comfort zone" gradually.

- Maintain a positive attitude and educate yourself about your back. This positive attitude has a beneficial effect on your healing. Remember most back pain resolves in two months. Don't assume you will be the exception.

Dr. B—

5

RECOGNIZING AND TREATING "MECHANICAL" LOW BACK PAIN

Most back pain is due to mechanical causes, such as muscle strain and trauma, disc degeneration and arthritis, herniated discs and sciatica, spinal stenosis and scoliosis. While my basic back pain relief program helps most back pain, it is important to know when you have a condition that may require more extensive medical treatment.

MUSCLE STRAIN, SPASM, AND TRAUMA

Back strain is injury to muscles, fascia, ligaments, or tendons and is one of the most common causes of low back pain. Everyday events cause back strain. You can cough or sneeze and cause this strain, or you can lift an object heavier than your muscles and ligaments can support. Or you can engage in a perfectly ordinary motion like bending over to pick up a sock.

Regardless of cause, the damage to the back tissues results in a reflex signal sent through the local nervous system, thereby alerting all the muscles supplied by the nerve that one of the stations in the network has been damaged. This alert protects the injured muscle and results in a muscle spasm, which tightens all the muscles in the network even though only one muscle was injured.

This muscle spasm in the lumbar spinal muscles is much like a charley horse that may develop when you run, ski, or swim. While severity varies, the pain can be overwhelming—you may have seen an Olympic runner actually fall to the ground as a result of a charley horse. Sometimes the muscle spasm is immobilizing and the person can't move at all. These muscle traumas are relatively common when bodies aren't well prepared for strenuous activity.

Ben, forty-two, came to see me with a typical winter story. A February snow-storm had dropped about eight inches of snow on his driveway, and he had to shovel it off before it hardened into ice. Because he played tennis in the summer months and walked on his treadmill during the winter, he thought he was in good shape. However, he did no weight lifting, and he went out to shovel the snow without warming up his muscles or wearing adequate outdoor clothing. Ten minutes into his shoveling job, he picked up a particularly heavy load of snow and twisted his body to the left to place it in a new pile. Before he could straighten his body, he felt severe pain in the right side of his low back, and the muscles in his back tightened as he stood there. With great effort, he managed to get into his house and get into bed, where, incidentally, his pain increased. The next day, Ben called to say that his back was so stiff he could not move. I told him to get out of bed and slowly and carefully walk around his house. Over time, Ben improved with a combination of exercises and nonprescription medications. However, this bout with pain made him promise himself that from then on, he would hire neighborhood kids to shovel his driveway.

Treatment

Muscle tightness may accompany any disorder that causes pain in the lumbar spine. Muscle spasms occur in order to reduce motion and decrease irritation to the injured structures, and the best way to relieve spasms is to keep mov-ing. Incremental—gradual—motions relieve spasm and allow the muscle to continuously test how far it can stretch. As the irritation is relieved, the mus-cles will go back to their normal tension. Remember this point, however: The first place to be injured will be the last to improve.

In addition to gradual motion, medications (aspirin-like medicines), cold packs (to relieve pain initially), a heating pad (to improve blood flow later), and stretching exercises are all appropriate self-care treatments to relieve the discomfort of back strain. Not all of these therapies are necessarily required, however, and you may respond to any one component (see chapter 4).

DISC DEGENERATION AND OSTEOARTHRITIS (LUMBAR SPONDYLOSIS)

After age thirty, your discs become less effective cushions; they start to resemble pancakes. In addition, loss of spacing puts more pressure on the facet joints at the back of the vertebrae, a process that results in lumbar spondylosis. These degenerative changes occur in all of us as we age, but in some of us they happen sooner.

Facet joints normally allow motion forward and backward and do not carry weight, but as the cushioning of the discs lessens, more and more body weight is placed on the facet joints. When the facet joints begin bearing weight, they start wearing out. These changes eventually lead to osteoarthritis, the most common form of arthritis; osteoarthritis often also involves the knee or hip.

Narrowing discs and changes in the facet joints may be a painless process, but it may also cause severe localized back pain. Individual differences are the rule, and we can't predict who will have pain associated with lumbar spondylosis. X rays and MRIs can detect changes in the joints and the degenerative discs, but these tests are unable to predict future pain. This is important because many patients come to me with MRIs demonstrating disc degeneration, but these changes may be inconsequential. As mentioned, a number of studies have shown that people with no complaints or history of back pain may show significant disc degeneration when given radiographic tests. On the other hand, osteoarthritis of the facet joints can cause significant back pain that requires attention in order to improve.

Almost everybody with lumbar spondylosis improves with nonsurgical therapy. Appliances—artificial discs—designed to replace discs in the spine remain in a developmental and experimental stage. We need many more years of testing before disc replacements will be available to the small group of patients with intractable back pain related to degenerative disc disease.

Treatment with Exercise and Medications

Disc degeneration and osteoarthritis are primarily treated with exercises. If you limit the motion of your spine, stiffness and fatigue often result. Range-of-motion exercises help maintain movement of the spine. Add medication if physical function is limited by increasing local back pain.

Osteoarthritis of the lumbar spine is treated with analgesics, NSAIDs, and muscle relaxants in varying combinations.

Facet Joint Injection for Osteoarthritis

If you have osteoarthritis, you will likely respond to oral drugs and will not need additional therapies. But you may be one of the few who have increased pain when bending to the side. The location of this side-bending pain does not change and is just off to the side of the middle of the back. These symptoms are characteristic of arthritis that affects the facet joints. When other therapies are ineffective, facet joint injections help decrease the pain.

The chance for success is increased when the injections are done with the help of X rays so that the needle can be placed exactly in the joint. Under fluoroscopic guidance, the injection of anesthetic and corticosteroid decreases the inflammation of the joint and the nerves supplying sensation to this area. The beneficial effect of the injection can last from days to months.

A more permanent, but more invasive, method to decrease pain in the facet joint is the use of heat (radiofrequency) or cold (cryoablation) to damage nerves supplying sensation to the facet joints. The point of the therapy is destruction of the nerves to the facet joint by searing or freezing them. We expect that the procedure will destroy all the nerves that cause the pain, without damaging any of the nerves supplying the muscles.

These procedures require you to be awake while the injections are given. Even when the procedure is done properly, all the sources of pain may not be reached. In addition, the procedure itself has the potential to cause increased low back pain. Therefore, I add these procedures as part of a complete prescription in only the most severe cases of facet syndrome that have been resistant to NSAIDs, muscle relaxants, exercises, and long-acting narcotics.

Osteoarthritis of the Hip

Arthritis of any type that affects the hip can cause groin pain. Nerves that supply sensation to the hip also innervate the muscles in the low back and thigh. Pain from the hip may also radiate down to the knee, and hip disease may show up as low back or thigh pain. If you have hip arthritis, you may have difficulty walking and you may attribute this to your back.

At fifty-five, Ellen, an attorney, had had difficulty walking for about six months. Her pain was localized to the right buttock and low back, and although she couldn't remember when her pain had started, she'd noticed a gradual increase in the severity of her symptoms. She had been to two other physicians who had focused attention on her lumbar spine as the cause of her symptoms, although X rays and an MRI scan of her spine did not reveal abnormalities. Despite lack of lumbar spine difficulties, her back pain increased and she had more and more trouble getting out of a chair or out of bed in the morning. Ellen's pain also had a detrimental effect on her sexual relationship with her husband because she had trouble finding a comfortable position during sex, one that did not cause more right buttock pain.

She had normal range of motion in her back, but when her right hip was moved by rotating her foot away from the center of her body, she experienced her "back" pain. An X ray taken of the pelvis, as opposed to the lumbar spine, revealed significant joint space narrowing and extra bone formation. When asked if she'd had trauma to this hip in the past, this limping lawyer remembered a horseback riding accident in which she had fallen on that hip but had only a bad bruise and no fracture. This old injury was the probable source of her current problems. I suggested treatment with exercises to strengthen her leg and anti-inflammatory medications. Currently, Ellen is walking without a limp, but she may be a candidate for hip replacement in the future.

HERNIATED DISC AND SCIATICA

In medical terms, a herniated disc is a rupture of the nucleus pulposus—the gel center—through the annulus fibrosus, the outer tire of the intervertebral discs (fig. 5.1). In popular language this is frequently referred to by the misnomer, "slipped disc." But discs do not slip. They herniate.

Most disc ruptures occur between the ages of thirty or forty, a time when discs contain a normal amount of gel and the outer tire is starting to wear out. The gel may remain inside the tire, which is a *disc protrusion*, or may escape outside the tire entirely, which is a *disc extrusion*. Extruded pieces of disc may move up or down the spinal canal, and discs may protrude to the front, the sides, or to the back (see fig. 5.1).

Protruded or extruded discs may not be painful unless they irritate the spinal nerves in the spinal canal. The body recognizes the abnormal position of the disc and tries to remove the abnormality. Inflammation that develops when the extruded piece of disc is recognized as "foreign tissue" in the spinal canal may be greater than inflammation that develops when there is a simple protrusion. The release of activated

NORMAL DISC

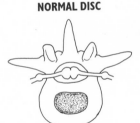

HERNIATED DISC

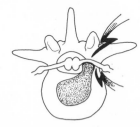

Figure 5.1 In a normal disc, the gel center stays in the center of the disc. In a herniated disc, the gel center has escaped from its covering and has invaded the spinal canal to compress the spinal nerve.

enzymes slowly dissolves the herniated portion of the disc, but may also inflame the nearby nerve. Once the nerve is inflamed, sciatica (radicular pain) is generated in the leg.

Sciatica caused by a herniated nucleus pulposus usually leads to leg pain that becomes worse with sitting and improved with standing or lying flat in bed with a pillow under the knees. In many instances, sciatica is preceded by a history of intermittent episodes of low back pain at which time the outer tire of the disc is stretched and under tension. Low back pain may decrease once the disc herniates because the outer tire is no longer under tension. Then low back pain is replaced with pain running to the leg and foot. This pain corresponds to the inflamed nerve caused by the gel from the disc pressing on the nerve.

Morning is the time of day most associated with increased forces on the disc because your discs absorb water during the night while you are lying flat. As mentioned in chapter 1, you are taller in the morning and shorter at the end of the day as gravity pushes water out of your discs, thereby making them thinner.

Any disc in the lumbar spine may rupture, but the ones at the bottom of the lumbar spine herniate most frequently because they carry a greater proportion of the weight of the body. Lumbar disc levels L-3, L-4, and L-5 each correspond to a nerve that affects a different part of your leg or foot. Knowing the part of the leg or foot that is numb or weak helps identify the location of the inflamed nerve.

- The L-3–L-4 level nerve runs to the thigh and affects the knee. L4 creates loss of sensation in front of your thigh and weakness in the front and back of your quadriceps, and loss of knee reflex.

- The L-4–L-5 level nerve runs to your big toe and involves sensation loss in front of your lower leg and big toe weakness, a foot drop from walking on your heel, but no loss of reflex.

- The L-5–S-1 level nerve affects the calf muscle and the bottom of the foot with weakness and loss of sensation from your calf to the outer three toes. There is reflex loss in your ankle.

These patterns are strongly correlated with the level of disc herniation and nerve compression. It is so characteristic that additional evaluation with X rays or an MRI is not necessary to initiate treatment for sciatica.

A progression of abnormalities in the nervous system corresponds to the inflamed nerve—from having no abnormalities to a loss of reflex and sensation to, finally, muscle weakness. You lose sensation before your leg becomes weak because the part of the nerve that attaches to muscles is deep inside the nerve and is surrounded on the outside by the sensory portion of the nerve. If you stretch your leg, the inflamed nerve causes pain down your leg. If you move your leg while lying flat, there will be a point where the affected nerve increases pain. In this flat position, bending your foot toward your head worsens the sciatica.

Pain is deep and sharp and progresses from the back downward in the involved leg, but sciatica may vary in intensity. You may experience pins and needles, or a burning sensation, typical to radicular pain. The pain may be so severe that your back is "locked," or just a dull ache that increases with movement. Pain worsens when you bend forward and improves with bending backward. Characteristically, people with herniated discs have pain with sitting, driving, walking, coughing, sneezing, and having a bowel movement. They have great difficulty bending forward because tightness in the muscles limits motion. Walking is difficult because the affected leg will not move forward in a normal manner, and the leg seems unable to hold your weight.

A herniated disc at a higher level in the lumbar spine can also cause anterior thigh pain, and an evaluation with a physician who will listen to your problem is important. No one physician can take care of all the problems that are associated with anterior thigh pain. However, your physician should be able to identify the general category of the problem and refer you to another physician with the expertise to evaluate and treat your disorder.

Herniated Disc: Treatment Without Surgery

Many studies report a good outcome with nonsurgical medical therapy in 80 percent or more of people with a herniated disc who are followed for five years. The primary element of treatment is movement, although for the first several days after the onset of sciatica, bed rest may be necessary to decrease pain.

Lying flat on your back with a pillow under your legs or resting on your side with a pillow placed between your legs takes tension off the inflamed nerve and decreases pressure on the herniated disc. As soon as possible, however, you should start walking on a flat surface. Stairs must be done with extreme care because of leg weakness.

Drug therapy in the form of anti-inflammatory drugs, muscle relaxants, and narcotics are helpful. The NSAIDs are a mainstay of therapy for acute herniated discs with nerve compression because of their anti-inflammatory and analgesic properties. The inflammation involving the nerve is a major cause of leg pain; NSAIDs decrease inflammation surrounding the disc and nerve, thereby reducing pain.

Hal, forty-five, a Washington lobbyist, told me his pain started when he lifted some heavy luggage after a business trip. Within two days he developed back pain that started to radiate into his left thigh. He then noticed an area of numbness over the top of his thigh and a slight imbalance when he went up or down the stairs. His examination revealed normal muscle strength, loss of pinprick sensation over the front of the thigh, the loss of the L-4 reflex at the knee, and pain that ran down the front of the thigh with raising the leg, a positive straight leg raising test.

Hal's exam was consistent with a disc herniation at the L-3–L-4 level, with impingement of the L-4 nerve root on the left. Hal had the option of an MRI scan, but I suggested that the scan would not alter the recommended therapy at the initial stage of this disorder, unless he developed greater weakness. He was pleased to hear that an MRI scan was not necessary, since he seemed to blanche at the idea of getting into the close quarters of the scanner.

Hal was treated with a combination of Voltaren XR (an NSAID) twice a day, prednisone (a corticosteroid), and oxycodone (a narcotic) up to four pills per day for pain, and an extension exercise program. Within ten days, his back and thigh pain started to improve. His reflex took about eight weeks to return, and his numbness took about three months to resolve. Gradually Hal stopped his medications; first his narcotic pain relievers, then the prednisone, and finally the Voltaren. At five months he had minimal pain in his back if he stood for an extended period.

Herniated Disc: Indications for Surgery

In certain cases, surgery to remove the portion of the disc that is pressing on the nerve may be indicated. However, indications for surgery are not always clear-cut, which makes the decision difficult for many people. For the rare person with loss of bladder or bowel function (cauda equina compression syndrome, or CEC) associated with a large disc herniation, surgery is the only choice.

The other indication for early surgery is progressive muscle weakness. If your foot is in a dropped position and cannot be raised, or the thigh muscle will not contract, surgical intervention must be considered. While you may recover from this situation, the process may take an extended period of time. Factors that play a role in the decision process include your pain tolerance, emotional response, work demands, and other lifestyle issues.

Remember the following statement that applies to the vast majority of people with back pain: *Lumbar spine disc surgery is done for leg pain, not back pain.* This statement is important because lumbar spine surgery relieves compression on nerves causing sciatica, leg pain. The surgery is done in the lumbar spine, and no matter what technique is used, the lumbar spine is injured during surgery.

Once the compression is removed, sciatica will resolve. If the appropriate disc level has been decompressed, the pain resolves quickly, with numbness improving over a longer period of time. What surgery often does is make an intolerable condition tolerable (see chapter 10).

CRACKED VERTEBRAL BODIES (SPONDYLOLYSIS AND SPONDYLOLISTHESIS)

Cartilage plates allow for the growth of bone while we are young, and one such plate exists in the lamina of the vertebrae between the joints. As we mature, our bones become solid and these cartilage plates close. Spondylolysis and spondylolisthesis occur because of a crack in this back section of a vertebra.

If physical activities during childhood, such as gymnastics, which involves bending backwards, cause enough strain on this cartilage plate, the plate will not close. This is a *spondylolysis*. If enough strain is placed on the cartilage plate, then the front end of the vertebra, which is no longer attached to the back part of the vertebra, may move forward, and that instability is a *spondylolisthesis*, commonly known as a slipped vertebra (see fig. 5.2). This instability occurs most frequently at the L-5 interspace. Because these spinal abnormalities occur during active growth during childhood, they are called *developmental spondylolisthesis*. For some, this instability remains painless throughout life. Even physically active individuals, such as football players, may remain free of pain. You may be unaware of the presence of a spondylolisthesis, but it may be identified by chance when an X ray is taken of the abdomen or spine for another reason.

Another form of spondylolisthesis occurs as we age and develops because the facet joints change their shape. This means that the facet joints can't keep the spine in its normal position, and therefore these joints allow slippage forward or backward. This problem, called *degenerative spondylolisthesis*, is a form of spinal osteoarthritis and occurs most commonly at L-4.

SPONDYLOLISTHESIS

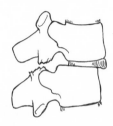

Figure 5.2 Spondylolisthesis—a break in the vertebra allows forward slippage.

Symptoms

Lumbar spondylolisthesis is characterized by an unstable spine. The front of the spine, the vertebral body, does not attach to the back of the spine, the facet joints. In most people the ligaments and muscles support the spine without abnormal motion. However, some people have abnormal movement of the spine with standing and they feel better in a forward posture. Back pain, with or without leg pain, occurs as the slippage becomes more significant, at which point you need to limit heavy lifting; therapy includes bracing and strengthening exercises.

Spondylolisthesis presents fewer symptoms while you sit and more pain when you stand, and generally the hamstring muscles are tight. In severe spondylolisthesis, an indentation in the lower lumbar spine is visible.

Treatment

Usually, spondylolysis does not require therapy. However, when necessary, symptomatic spondylolisthesis can be treated with flexion exercises (bending forward), bracing to support the spine, and anti-inflammatory medications to decrease pain. When bracing is unable to control pain, lumbar spine surgery (bony fusion) is necessary, but this is rare. This operation can be very useful to the younger spondylolisthesis patients with persistent low back pain (see chapter 10).

PIRIFORMIS SYNDROME

The piriformis muscle is located deep inside the buttock. The muscle has its origin on the sacral vertebrae and stretches to insert on the thighbone. The muscle works to rotate the thigh laterally. The sciatic nerve runs under the piriformis muscle as it leaves the spinal canal and goes through the sciatic notch and travels down the leg.

Any disorder that irritates the piriformis muscle will cause it to contract, thereby compressing the sciatic nerve. This compression causes a diffuse pain down the leg that follows no single nerve. This characteristic differentiates piriformis syndrome from nerve compression associated with a herniated disc. With piriformis syndrome, you may have difficulty walking because of leg pain. Women may experience vaginal and pelvic pain during sexual intercourse. The pain is made worse when the muscle is stretched, as in bringing the bent leg across the center of the body.

Electrodiagnostic tests will document nerve compression in the area of the buttock, and an MRI scan may detect an enlarged muscle inside the pelvis.

Therapy includes stretching exercises, analgesics, anti-inflammatory medications, and muscle relaxants. With persistent pain, injections of local anesthetics and corticosteroids in the muscles may help (see chapter 7).

SPINAL STENOSIS

As the space in the spinal canal decreases, more compression is placed on the nerves within the canal. This results in narrowing (stenosis). Disc degeneration and osteoarthritis of the lumbar spine cause a decrease in the room inside the spinal canal. Some fortunate people are born with larger spinal canals, but others have canals with a shape that from an early age diminishes the volume in the spine.

Structures that take up room in the spinal canal include extra bone around the joints (osteophytes), degenerative discs, and folded ligaments that line the interior of the spinal canal (ligamentum flavum). Lumbar stenosis may occur in the center or side of the spinal canal or the foramen opening for the nerve root. These areas of spinal canal compression are correlated with pain in different locations in the legs:

- Central stenosis causes pain in one or both legs with walking.
- Lateral stenosis causes pain down one leg with standing.
- Stenosis of a neural foramen causes leg pain that is persistent, regardless of the position.

Decreased arterial blood flow to the leg (vascular claudication) must be differentiated from leg pain that is secondary to spinal stenosis. Vascular claudication, which is one of the important symptoms of cardiovascular disease, causes leg pain with activity such as walking or running. Standing without walking does not cause pain with vascular claudication.

Pain associated with spinal stenosis may cause back, buttock, thigh, lower leg, or foot pain. The pain may come in any combination of locations from the low back to the foot. You may feel pain only in your leg and none in your back. In addition to pain, you may also have numbness, unusual sensations like tingling (paresthesias), and weakness in the lower extremities. People with spinal stenosis are able to ride a stationary bicycle or walk up stairs or an incline without difficulty. However, standing or walking down the stairs or down an incline causes pain. Spinal stenosis causes leg pain while walking or standing because this posture causes a narrowing of the volume of the spinal canal and stops the blood flow to the spinal nerves. This posture may cause direct pressure on the nerves by structures in the canal including joints, ligaments, or discs. When you bend forward or sit down, your posture increases the volume in the canal, and restores blood flow to the nerve.

Because stenosis can occur at multiple levels of the spine, and more than one level may be causing your leg pain, careful correlation between your symptoms and radiographic findings is essential to determine the critical areas of stenosis. This is the time where electrodiagnostic testing may be helpful in separating central from peripheral nerve disorders, as well as determining the level of central nerve involvement.

Sometimes symptoms of lumbar spinal stenosis are unusual. Early in my medical career, Evan, sixty-four, came to see me with one of the most unusual requests I've encountered. An executive with a large corporation, Evan was despondent because his physical ailment was having a detrimental effect on his marriage, and he wanted me to quickly diagnose and treat his problem— and save his marriage!

His problem started about a year prior to his office visit. While standing, he had increasing pain in his right knee, which was relieved when he sat down. A number of physicians had examined his knee, but no abnormality appeared on X rays and MRI scans of his knee. Physical therapy and knee braces for support had no effect.

So, how were his knee problems relevant to his marriage? Not only did Evan work hard, he played hard, too, and he played squash three times a week without any significant pain in his knee. But if his wife wanted to dance with him, his turn on the dance floor lasted only three or four minutes because of pain in his knee. Naturally, his wife didn't understand how he could play squash for hours on end but could not dance for more than four minutes. She suspected an affair! Evan assured me that he loved his wife and was not fooling around.

The answer to the executive's problem showed up in his history. When he played squash, he was bent forward, a position that relieves spinal stenosis. When he was dancing, he was standing, an extended posture that increases the symptoms of spinal stenosis. When I examined him, his knee was normal, but when I asked him to stand in an extended posture for a few minutes, his knee pain returned, and when he sat down, his knee pain resolved. But an MRI of his lumbar spine revealed spinal stenosis, and a course of NSAIDS and epidural corticosteroid injections improved his condition. Soon, Evan was able to play squash *and* dance with his wife. He believed his diagnosis saved his marriage.

Evan's case is an example of a situation in which physical examination does not reveal a problem unless you exercise until the symptoms appear. At that time sensory, muscle, and reflex changes may become abnormal, but these abnormal findings reverse when back and leg pain resolve. Plain X rays of the lumbar spine may demonstrate degenerative disc disease with facet joint narrowing, but they may not explain the symptoms you experience. MRI scans can be helpful in identifying the location of nerve impingement. CT scans are even better than MRI's at visualizing the bony changes associated with spinal stenosis.

Regardless of test results, the correlation between symptoms and anatomic changes is not as closely associated in spinal stenosis as it is with herniated discs. This has important implications for the role of surgery in the treatment of spinal stenosis.

Spinal Stenosis: Treatment Without Surgery

Treatment of spinal stenosis starts with becoming educated about the mechanics of the spine and the way your symptoms increase and decrease with this condition. You will understand why you like to bend over the shopping cart in the supermarket and avoid leg pain. Symptoms of spinal stenosis are improved if you sit down, but you can't sit all the time. This is where drug therapy comes in, because it can help improve function.

NSAIDs help treat the pain of osteoarthritis, which is the major cause of spinal stenosis, and these medications are able to decrease swelling in the facet joints as well as the soft tissues in the spinal canal, but there is risk of stomach ulcers. Newer medications, the COX-2 inhibitors, may be particularly helpful to older osteoarthritis patients who are at risk of developing ulcers. (See chapter 7 for more on these medications.)

Epidural corticosteroid injections may be helpful for leg pain associated with spinal stenosis. However, the sequence of injections is different for spinal stenosis than for herniated disc because the underlying abnormalities are different. With a herniated disc, the acute inflammatory response acts on soft tissues (the gel in the disc) that are herniated. The inflammatory reaction can remove the herniated portion of the disc. At the same time, the inflammatory response irritates the spinal nerve. In order to control the inflammation over a short period of time, epidurals are given as three injections in a short period of time.

I call sixty-eight-year-old Betty "the woman who rode around the world on her bike." Betty had significant spinal stenosis at multiple levels, and an orthopedic surgeon had said that a multilevel operation would be necessary to open the levels that were compressing her nerves and causing leg pain that limited her walking to about two blocks. Betty did not want surgery because she was unsure which level was the most important in controlling her pain. Instead, she chose to have epidural corticosteroid injections when her symptoms required. This meant an injection every four to six months for about twelve years. When she didn't have the injections, she again had difficulty walking two blocks, but with the injections she could get to her health club for regular workouts. Although limited in the standing position, she was quite functional in the seated position, so she rode on a stationary bicycle at least four days a week on a regular basis. Her particular health club counted up her miles, and once she passed the 25,000 mile mark, she was given an "around the world" award, and naturally she wanted to show it to me.

You will be unable to have injections if you are taking blood thinners for clotted blood vessels or artificial heart valve difficulties. Low doses of prednisone rather than epidural injections may work. In older people, corticosteroids are more toxic and should be used only if the drug has a significant beneficial effect on function. If older people are able to get around and are not forced into social isolation because of back and leg pain, the risk-benefit ratio of low-dose corticosteroids favors the drug.

Spinal Stenosis: Indications for Surgery

When pain constantly interferes with walking or leg pain occurs immediately with standing, surgery to remove the stenosis is appropriate. If a single level of stenosis is present and correlates with the reported symptoms, surgical outcome tends to be good. Greater difficulty occurs when multiple levels of stenosis are present and clinical symptoms are diffuse throughout the leg. In these circumstances, an experienced surgeon can complete an appropriate preoperative evaluation to determine the extent of lumbar spine surgery that is required to improve leg pain (see chapter 10).

SCOLIOSIS

Scoliosis is a lateral curvature of the spine that forms an "S" shape (see fig. 2.1, page 36), the cause of which is unknown in most cases. The spine may also twist like a corkscrew (rotatory scoliosis). Minor curvatures of the spine are common and usually aren't associated with pain or dysfunction.

Although adults get it, scoliosis is most often associated with teenage girls, and some schools now sponsor screening programs that identify at-risk teenagers at an early stage of curvature. Several factors suggest an early scoliosis is developing: one shoulder higher than another, an uneven hemline, the prominence of one shoulder blade compared to the other. When scoliosis is detected early, exercise and a brace may help to avoid surgery later in life. Adults, primarily women, may develop the condition between ages twenty and forty. Most curvatures are stable and do not progress with age. In older people spinal curvature may develop when disc space narrows and spinal joints deform.

Recognizing and Treating "Mechanical" Low Back Pain

When younger people develop severe curvatures (over forty degrees), slow spontaneous progression of the deformity results. The imbalance in the spine may also be related to leg length inequalities, when one leg is shorter than the other. However, many such differences are of little consequence, and we don't yet know what degree of difference in leg length is linked with low back pain. A heel lift under the short leg is beneficial in some cases. Progressive curvature has consequences, and vital organs in the chest and abdomen may be squeezed.

Noncritical curvatures are treated with exercises and medications. Young people with severe scoliosis require the placement of metal rods (called Harrington rods) that lengthen the spine and reduce the curvature. Only experienced surgeons should do this operation.

The Mother With Rods

Sonja complained of increasing low back pain after sitting for long periods at her computer. Now forty-five, she had had scoliosis as a teenager, and because bracing had not worked and the spinal curve was severe, Harrington rods were placed in her spine. She had given birth to two children without difficulty, but now her work required long stints at the computer. She was concerned that her curve was getting worse and her rods were wearing out.

When I examined Sonja, I found that her curve was no worse than it was at the time the rods were first placed. However, the pressure of the rods themselves can place more pressure on the discs and joints of the vertebrae where the clips attach to the spine. She had developed some arthritis at these sites, and range of motion exercises were needed, along with daily nonsteroidal medication. She also joined an aquaerobics (water exercise) program and she swims three times a week. This combination therapy allows her to live normally and do her computer work with minimal discomfort.

Sonja's story helps dispel the misconception that having scoliosis surgery means limited motion and a limited life. In fact, most scoliosis patients can lead normal lives, including having children if they choose, as long as their problem is identified in a timely manner.

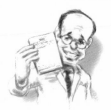

DR. B'S PRESCRIPTION SUMMARY
R⟲

- Back strain is a muscle injury of the low back. Keep moving as much as you can tolerate.

- Disc narrowing is part of the natural aging process that can cause back pain. Flexion (bending forward) exercises help decrease pain and keep you moving.

- Arthritis in your hip can cause pain that is located in your lower back.

- Disc herniations cause back and leg pain made worse with sitting. Sciatica can resolve with extension exercises (bending backward), and oral or injected medications. Disc surgery is required for muscle weakness or intractable pain

- Spinal stenosis causes leg pain made worse with walking or standing. Non-surgical therapy helps the ability to walk longer distances. Surgery improves the condition but does not keep the problem from returning.

- When the "S" curve of scoloiosis is severe, it can cause back pain.

Dr. B—

6

RECOGNIZING AND TREATING MEDICAL CAUSES OF LOW BACK PAIN

Many medical illnesses can cause low back pain. Diabetics with nerve damage, for example, feel pain in their back as well as other areas. An undetected bone tumor or cancer can be the cause of back pain. So can problems in nearby organs such as the kidneys or gastrointestinal system. In general, low back pain from a medical condition progresses slowly and persists despite the basic care program. You will also have one of the red flag symptoms mentioned in chapter 1, such as fever or weight loss. It's important that you and your doctor treat the underlying illness, not just the back pain.

INFECTION

Persistent fever and/or weight loss that accompanies back pain can be infection or a tumor of the spine. Bacterial infections may affect the bone (osteomyelitis), disc (discitis), or joint (septic arthritis). The source of the bacteria may be an infection in the skin, urinary tract, oral cavity, or any penetrating wound. Between 1 and 2 percent of people undergoing spinal surgery develop an infection at the surgical site. Some are at increased risk for infections. Diabetics may have decreased immunity to infection because of low antibody levels, as do AIDS (acquired immunodeficiency syndrome) patients. Drug users may use unsterile needles, which allow bacteria to enter the bloodstream, and these bacteria may migrate to the spine and cause pain.

Pain caused by an infection progresses slowly but becomes severe. It is present during rest and exacerbated by movement. An infection is diagnosed by taking a culture of the organism, either from drawn blood or from the infected area in the spine, which requires placing a needle into the area of infection. Once the bacterium is identified, the infection is treated with specific antibiotics that will kill the organism. It may be necessary to drain the area if antibiotics alone are insufficient. The longer it takes to detect the infection, the more likely it is that surgical drainage will be necessary.

BONE TUMORS AND CANCER

Cancer that involves the lumbar spine can cause loss of appetite, and even before back pain begins, weight loss may occur. Once pain appears, however, it generally progresses rapidly. Cancers affecting the lumbar spine usually originate in other organs, such as the prostate in men and the breast in women. Multiple myeloma, a bone marrow cancer, is the most common cancer originating in the spinal tissues.

Blood tests may indicate the presence of a tumor. Plain X rays may not identify the location of the tumor, and a bone scan is a sensitive but nonspecific test for identifying bone lesions. MRI and CT scans best identify bony and soft tissue tumor involvement. When a tumor is diagnosed, a biopsy or total removal of the tumor is done, depending on the type, location, and size.

Bone tumors—benign or malignant—of the spinal column or spinal cord are the primary concern in people who have pain at night or when lying flat. Pain results when an expanding tumor and associated inflammation compress the spinal nerves. Although we don't know why, some benign tumors of the spine are more painful at night than during the day.

MRI is the most sensitive method to detect bony abnormalities, spinal cord compression, and soft tissue involvement of tumorlike (neoplastic) lesions. The abnormal tissue is examined under the microscope to determine if it is benign or malignant. Therapy depends on the outcome of the diagnostic evaluation. Total removal of the tumor is always preferred as long as vital tissues are not sacrificed.

Dennis, a twenty-four-year-old salesperson, thought at first that his yearlong nighttime back pain was related to the fact that he slept in a different bed every night while on the road. Eventually he realized that the beds were not the problem. Dennis's pain increased at night, but aspirin significantly diminished it when he was at home in his own bed. Once he stopped taking aspirin the pain came back.

Plain X rays of his spine showed a lesion in the L-3 vertebra. A bone scan was "hot" (increased bone activity) over the same area without any additional areas of involvement in the remainder of the skeleton. A CT scan identified the exact location of the lesion, and because Dennis was tired of taking aspirin on a daily basis, he had the lesion removed. It was an *osteoid osteoma*, a benign bone tumor, so its removal was all that was required to eliminate Dennis's back pain.

INFLAMMATORY DISEASES

If morning back stiffness lasts an hour or less, it is probably caused by a mechanical disorder. When it lasts several hours, it would indicate inflammatory arthritis of the spine, or *spondyloarthropathy*. Inflammatory arthritis of the spine causes the proteins and white cells that fight infection in the bloodstream to attack spinal structures. The lining of the joints, the synovium, swells and impedes motion. With spondyloarthropathies, the body responds to inflammation by depositing calcium in the inflamed tissues. The end result is a spine that has fused facet joints and calcified ligaments.

Rheumatoid arthritis (RA) is a common inflammatory arthritis, but it does not affect the lumbar spine. RA affects most joints in the arms and legs and the cervical spine, but for reasons not yet understood, it spares the lower portion of the spine.

Psoriatic arthritis does cause back pain. Up to 7 percent of people with psoriasis, a common skin disease, also develop this form of arthritis. Most have the skin lesions either prior to or at the same time that the arthritis appears, although a small number have characteristic arthritis symptoms but no evidence of skin abnormalities. Arthritis may be present for ten to twenty years before the psoriatic skin lesions appear.

These conditions and others such as ankylosing spondylitis (AS), Reiter's syndrome, and inflammatory bowel disease (IBD) arthritis cause inflammation of the spine (spondylitis).

AS and Reiter's syndrome are more frequent in men, while psoriatic and IBD spondylitis occur with equal frequency in men and women. AS occurs in 1 percent of the U.S. population; Reiter's syndrome is the most common cause of arthritis in young adult men. Psoriatic arthritis occurs in 0.1 percent of the general population.

Bilateral sacroiliac joint pain is associated with AS and IBD arthritis and is the initial location for joint inflammation. Reiter's syndrome and psoriatic spondylitis may have unilateral sacroiliac joint pain and stiffness or may affect the lumbar spine without involving the sacroiliac joints. AS may affect only the sacroiliac joints or may extend through the entire length of the spine to the cervical spine. AS is not a disease only of joints but is frequently accompanied with severe eye inflammation (iritis), which can lead to blindness if left untreated. In a very few AS patients, the aortic valve of the heart may become leaky and require replacement. IBD arthritis occurs in people with ulcerative colitis and Crohn's disease. The spondyloarthropathy in these patients has similar characteristics to that of AS.

Symptoms of Reiter's syndrome include superficial eye inflammation (conjunctivitis), inflammation of the urinary tract (urethritis), and arthritis affecting the spine and lower extremity joints. Reiter's syndrome may also include fever, weight loss, and afternoon fatigue. A characteristic skin rash affects the palms and soles and also the tip of the penis. Painless oral ulcers also occur in a few people with Reiter's syndrome. Occasionally victims of salmonella and shigella epidemics (usually occurring in restaurants and fast food chains) will develop Reiter's syndrome.

Chlamydia trachomatis, an organism infecting the urinary tract, is linked with the onset of Reiter's syndrome. (Chlamydia infection is a sexually transmitted disease.) Reiter's patients may develop the whole syndrome of symptoms and signs, including gastrointestinal and urinary symptoms, even if the initial infection occurred in another organ system.

The Unfortunate Conventioneer

Sidney, thirty, was attending a business convention in the Far East and had unprotected sex with a woman he knew, but whom he had not seen for a number of years. After returning home, he developed fever, gastrointestinal symptoms including diarrhea, and mild pain over his heel. (Heel pain is inflammation of the attachment of tendons to bone, a common location for Reiter's syndrome inflammation.) Over the next two weeks, Sidney had an episode of conjunctivitis and increasing knee pain. When his primary doctor saw him, Sidney did not mention his sexual encounter or any urinary symptoms, and an evaluation for a gastrointestinal disorder was negative. Only after he developed pain with urination and a rash on his penis did the possibility of Reiter's syndrome arise. Sidney developed most of the symptoms of the disorder over the next three months.

Sidney's diagnosis was genitourinary chlamydia infection, and he was treated with a course of antibiotics and one of the new COX-2 inhibitors because of a past history of ulcers that increased his risk of bleeding when taking aspirin. After six weeks, all his symptoms except his knee pain were gone, and Sidney still takes a COX-2 inhibitor to control his knee pain.

Sidney's case illustrates the confusion that can arise when the source of the initial infection is overlooked. Always be truthful with your physician about your entire history, including your sexual history. Sidney also illustrates one of the consequences of having unprotected sex. It is entirely possible that Sidney's partner did not know she carried the chlamydia infection, because it may not produce overt symptoms.

Finding Spondyloarthropathy

Spondyloarthropathy causes stiffness in all directions of spinal motion and tenderness over inflamed portions of the spine. X rays of the lumbosacral spine help to identify early changes of the arthritis, including loss of lumbar curve (lordosis), erosion in the sacroiliac joints, and squaring of vertebral bodies. The front of the vertebral body has an indentation running from the top to the bottom. When a vertebral body is squared, inflammation erodes the prominent part of the top and bottom of the curve. The vertebral body becomes a square.

We do not need to use the more costly radiographic tests to identify the skeletal abnormalities of spondylitis. Histocompatibility testing, a blood test, identifies genetic factors that predispose people to develop spondyloarthropathy. HLA-B27 is a marker associated with these illnesses but does not by itself cause the illness. Approximately 8 percent of the Caucasian U.S. population is B27 positive and does not have a spondyloarthropathy. A total of 2 percent of all HLA-B27 positive Caucasians have AS.

Treatment

Treatment for the spondyloarthropathies includes range of motion and deep breathing exercises; NSAIDs decrease inflammation and facilitate motion but do not cure the disease or prevent calcification. Antibiotic therapy for Reiter's syndrome is most useful early in the course of the illness. Topical therapy for psoriatic skin disease may have a beneficial effect on joint inflammation. Control of IBD may also prove beneficial for joint symptoms.

Anti-inflammatory Diets

My patients often ask me if diet has any effect on their low back pain. Only about 10 percent of low back pain is caused by an inflammatory disorder like arthritis, and diets that may decrease inflammation have the potential to help the small number with chronic inflammatory lumbar spine conditions.

Fasting diets affect immune function that mediates inflammatory disorders, but this is highly variable and controversial. Fasting for certain periods of time may decrease inflammatory disorders like rheumatoid arthritis through a mechanism of malnutrition that suppresses the body's defense mechanisms. However, the stress of fasting may actually stimulate the immune system. Immune status is also affected by the extent of the fast, whether it is a total or partial fast. In any case, fasting must be closely monitored.

Food sensitivities can also stimulate the immune response. The gastrointestinal tract in people who develop arthritis may allow certain foods that usually would not be absorbed, such as the proteins in cow's milk, to enter the body. When this happens, the body responds by producing antibodies to signal increased immune response that may be associated with joint, muscle, or blood vessel inflammation. Experimentation with elimination diets has suggested that removing eggs, milk, chocolate, wheat, beans, and shellfish from the diet may be helpful.

Vegetarian diets, supplemented with nuts, eggs, and dairy products (unless sensitivities to these foods are present), along with antioxidants and B vitamins, may also decrease joint inflammation. In general, reducing animal fats in the diet and taking antioxidant supplements may decrease the level of inflammation.

Eliminating foods from the diet to control pain and inflammation may not be as helpful as *adding* certain foods. For example, consuming cold-water fish such as salmon and mackerel may help decrease inflammation. The connection between fish and inflammation has to do with the fats in the membranes of our cells. These membrane fats are the sources of the chemicals that produce prostaglandins (PG), which are one of the factors that promote inflammation and pain. Fish oils, specifically the omega-3 family of polyunsaturated fatty acids (EPA, DHA), are different from human oils (arachidonic acid). The prostaglandins formed with fish oils are less inflammatory than those formed with arachidonic acid. When you consume cold-water fish, you can replace the fats in the membranes of your cells with fish oils. This in turn results in less inflammation and pain.

Any of these diets takes time to work. In addition, it is necessary to implement a significant substitution before anti-inflammatory effects occur. Fish oil supplements may hasten this substitution, but amounts of three to five grams per day may be necessary to obtain the beneficial effect. You may need to consume so much omega-3 fatty acid that you may start taking on a fishy aroma.

Plant sources of special fatty acids such as gamma linolenic acid (GLA) include flaxseed, evening primrose, and borage oils. These sources of fatty acids also produce prostaglandins that are less inflammatory. A significant amount of these plant oils are needed on a daily basis to achieve an anti-inflammatory effect. The problem with some of these plant and fish fatty acids is that they contain calories. A consultation with a physician or nutritionist would result in a diet that includes these fatty acids while maintaining a reasonable daily calorie intake.

DISH SYNDROME
(DIFFUSE IDIOPATHIC SKELETAL HYPEROSTOSIS)

DISH syndrome affects the spine and is sometimes confused with AS. It is different from AS because the sacroiliac joints are unaffected while the front of the spine is altered, leaving the facet joints untouched. The two disorders are often confused because DISH, like AS, causes calcification of the spine. DISH occurs most commonly in Caucasian men fifty and older, compared to AS, which often affects people in their twenties. DISH may be asymptomatic and often is detected only on X rays.

Morning stiffness and decreased range of motion usually lasts an hour or less, and back pain is higher in the spine near the thorax. No organ systems other than the bone and joints are affected, and HLA-B27 is negative in DISH patients. X rays of the spine show flowing calcifications (resembling candle wax) on the anterior portion of at least four thoracic vertebrae. The lumbar spine is affected less frequently.

Treatment for DISH involves movement (strongly recommended) and deep breathing exercises. No therapy exists that removes the calcifications in the spine, and surgical removal is not appropriate.

OCHRONOSIS

This is another rare and unusual illness that may be confused with AS. Ochronosis is caused by the accumulation of a chemical, homogentisic acid, in tissues. Over time, this accumulated chemical becomes black, and the deposits blacken many areas, including the ears and the whites of the eyes. The chemical is also passed in the urine, thereby making it black if it is exposed to the sun. The same chemical settles in the tissues around the spine and causes calcifications that mimic AS. No effective therapy exists. Fortunately, ochronosis is extremely rare, occuring in about 1 in 10 million people.

FIBROMYALGIA

Fibromyalgia (FM) is a soft tissue pain syndrome characterized by chronic pain in discrete tender point areas, including the lumbar spine; but it is not associated with any structural abnormalities of muscle, bone, or cartilage. The persistent pain and chronic fatigue associated with the illness prevent those who have it from achieving their full potential. It also brings with it tension headaches, irritable bowel syndrome, and low blood pressure.

Although controversy exists about the existence of FM, about 15 percent of people who visit a rheumatologist satisfy the criteria for this disorder. Women, particularly young and middle-aged women, are affected more frequently than men. In about half the cases, the onset of FM seems to follow an injury, excessive physical activity, or emotional or psychological stress. The pain may be unremitting with durations of up to twenty years, or the discomfort may be migratory and wax and wane.

Fatigue is also a prominent feature of FM, and these patients often report restless sleep and morning exhaustion. Cold or humid weather, overactivity, total inactivity, stress, menses, and poor sleep exacerbate FM. Symptoms improve with moderate activity; warm, dry weather; and massage.

Areas that are tender to palpation are referred to as tender points and are localized, most commonly to the upper border of the shoulders, knees, elbows, and the lumbar spine. There is no pain outside the area. There may be twelve or more sensitive areas in someone with primary FM. Other than identifying these tender points, a physical examination usually is normal. The diagnosis of FM is based on eliminating other conditions.

The American College of Rheumatology in 1990 reported classification criteria for FM that includes a history of widespread pain for a minimum of three months (pain in four body quadrants) and pain in eleven of eighteen tender points when manually palpated. In addition, the presence of another disorder does not exclude a diagnosis of FM. In a study involving patients who'd had spinal surgery and who were referred to a spine center for lumbar pain, 12 percent had FM complicating their condition, but the FM had remained undiagnosed.

Treatment of FM requires a multifaceted approach. In many circumstances, educating the patients about their illness is reassuring and relieves some symptoms. Most people are encouraged to know their symptoms are not "all in their head." Once they understand that their condition is not life threatening, deforming, or degenerating, even though it causes chronic pain, they can adjust their lifestyle.

Treatment

Rest and relaxation are important for FM patients who are overworked. We generally encourage you to remain at work if possible, while at the same time avoiding excessive fatigue. Range of motion and stretching exercises encourage improved muscle function, and an aerobic exercise program is also essential. Heat treatments are also useful.

NSAIDs help reduce FM-related pain. Tramadol (Ultram), a nonnarcotic analgesic, also may be helpful. To control localized pain, tender points can be injected with a combination of anesthetic agent and a long-acting corticosteroid.

Antidepressants such as the tricyclic Elavil (amitriptyline) and muscle relaxants like Flexeril (cyclobenzaprine) increase the brain's serotonin to influence mood. Increased levels of serotonin reduce pain and induce sleep. Drugs called selective serotonin re-uptake inhibitors (SSRIs) like Prozac (fluoxetine) or Zoloft (sertraline) may help certain people, but in general, this class of antidepressants does not work as effectively for FM as the tricyclic drugs.

The basic therapeutic program for FM involves a tricyclic agent, patient education, and aerobic exercise. Adding an NSAID is optional and depends on the patient's muscle pain. Injecting tender points is useful if they are few in number. Over the long term, compliance with the program is essential.

TENSION MYOSITIS SYNDROME

Generalized muscle tension in people with chronic anxiety and stress causes pain, and this phenomenon has been given a name: tension myositis syndrome (TMS). Dr. John Sarno, who popularized the TMS diagnosis, suggests that the autonomic nervous system, in response to repressed emotions like anxiety and anger, causes a decrease of blood flow to muscles, which results in oxygen deprivation, known as ischemia.

According to Dr. Sarno's proposition, ischemia is the reason for pain in muscles, tendons, and ligaments. Muscle tension is also thought to occur in a similar manner in FM. In this way, Sarno proposes that TMS and FM are similar disorders and treatment is psychological, not physical. If the repressed thoughts are removed, the pain will resolve.

Although I believe that the central nervous system plays a significant role in the response to pain, I do not agree with the hypothesis upon which TMS is based. I have had a number of patients with back strain or fibromyalgia who have not had any increase in muscle tension although they have been exquisitely sensitive at tender points, many of which are over ligaments or tendons, not muscles. In addition, when compared to muscles, ligaments and tendons require minimal amounts of oxygen to function. Ischemia would have a significantly different effect on these tissues.

Undoubtedly, chronic pain can make you anxious, but being anxious does not cause low back pain, which can be modified by changes in physical positions. As for therapy, I would agree with Dr. Sarno that physical activity is beneficial in restoring function. Resolving stressful issues is good for everyone, those with low back pain and those without it. To control chronic pain it is necessary to reduce anxiety and reverse fatigue. But, if you have AS (inflammation of the spine) for example, you can't expect your pain to go away just because you resolve your anger with your boss, or you change jobs, or you work through other stressful problems.

MYOFASCIAL PAIN SYNDROME

Low back pain is a common symptom of myofascial pain syndrome (MPS). Remember the fascia is that "plastic wrap" covering of your muscles. MPS is a regional pain syndrome with two major symptoms: a localized area of deep muscle tenderness (trigger point) accompanied by a palpable nodule in the muscle, and a specific area of referred pain distant from the trigger point.

Pressure over a trigger point creates a dull, aching pain in a referral pattern that does not follow any characteristic muscle structure. Although the symptoms may sound similar, FM and MPS are not the same illness. MPS is a localized pain syndrome with sudden onset and trigger points that radiate pain. Treatment for MPS involves injecting trigger points with anesthetics, along with the use of superficial cooling and muscle stretching.

OSTEOPOROSIS

Osteoporosis is most common in Caucasian postmenopausal women, but it also affects African American, Asian, and Hispanic women. Men cannot afford to be complacent, because they account for about 20 percent of osteoporosis cases. Ten million Americans have osteoporosis, with another 18 million at risk for fracture because of decreased bone mineral density. The primary locations for osteoporosis include the spine, hipbone, pelvis, and wrist.

Bone is made up of a framework of collagen that is like the girders of a building. A mineral compound containing calcium and phosphorus forms the cement that layers the girders. Just as our soft tissues are alive and always changing, bone is continuously being remodeled by cells that excavate (*osteoclasts*) and rebuild (*osteoblasts*). Our bones are a constant source of calcium for the bloodstream, which carries the calcium throughout the body in order to play its role in a number of normal functions, including muscle contraction. During our youth, calcium is absorbed and stored in bone, and the building cells, the osteoblasts, predominate. As we age, the excavating cells, osteoclasts, are more active, which results in calcium loss. If the calcium content becomes too low, the bone is weakened and is at risk for fracture.

Spinal pain localized in the middle of the back over the bone is associated with disorders that fracture or expand bone. Any systemic process that increases calcium loss from bone (osteoporosis), causes bone death (sickle cell anemia), or replaces bone cells with inflammatory or neoplastic cells (multiple myeloma) weakens vertebral bone to the point that fracture may occur spontaneously or with minimal trauma. Acute fractures create sudden onset of severe pain, but the pain may be the initial manifestation of the underlying disorder.

Primary risk factors for osteoporosis include: female sex, increased age, estrogen deficiency, family history of osteoporosis, white race, low body weight, smoking, and history of fractures. Osteoporosis may also occur as a secondary condition to medical disorders and medications such as long-term use of corticosteroids like prednisone. Normal hormonal changes that occur after menopause are linked with osteoporosis.

If fractures have occurred in the thoracic spine, a kyphosis—dowager's hump—may be present. This is an exaggerated forward curve of the thoracic spine that pushes the head forward. X rays may show alterations in the bone but do not reveal small fractures. A bone scan can detect increased bone activity soon after a fracture occurs, and a CT scan may identify the abnormality. However, locating the lesion is not enough to allow us to determine the specific cause of the bony changes.

Available therapies include estrogens, selective estrogen receptor modulators (SERM), bisphosphonates, salmon calcitonin, and fluorides. All of these therapies have benefits but carry risk of toxicity, too. Discuss your individual choices with your physician, but don't put it off; the time to reverse the effects of osteoporosis is now.

The best treatment is still prevention. See chapter 11 for more information.

BLOOD DISORDERS AND ANEURYSMS

Hemoglobin is the protein that carries oxygen to our tissues, and if the proteins making up hemoglobin develop abnormalities, their ability to carry oxygen to tissues is compromised. Red blood cells also may change shape, which then impedes flow in the small blood vessels. Hemoglobinopathies are a group of blood disorders that cause abnormalities of the hemoglobin that packs the red cells in our blood. The primary example is sickle cell anemia. When oxygen levels are low, red blood cells will lose their normal shape and become sickled. Sickled cells will clog small blood vessels throughout the body, which is part of what we call a sickle cell crisis. The spinal vertebrae are primary locations for this blood vessel change. Lack of oxygen causes death of tissues, in this case, bone tissue. Bone death (avascular necrosis) is readily apparent on X rays of the lumbar spine.

No therapy currently is available to reverse the single amino acid substitution that results in the abnormal hemoglobin. In the future, the ability to substitute normal genetic code for abnormal codes will offer the cure for this illness. Until that time, sickle cell patients are treated with intravenous fluids, pain medications, and oxygen.

Aneurysms

Throbbing pain may occur in your low back with an aneurysm of the abdominal aorta. The aorta is the major arterial blood vessel that supplies blood from the heart to the rest of the body and runs just in front of the lumbar spine. An aneurysm is a weakening in the wall of the vessel, and is analogous to weakening in the sidewall of a tire. As the tire weakens, the remaining wall experiences increasing pressure. If the pressure becomes too great, the tire may blow out. Similarly, if the pressure on the wall of the vessel occurs, then an aneurysm will rupture.

There may be no symptoms with a slowly growing aneurysm, but vascular changes may be noted on X rays of the abdomen taken for other reasons. Pain frequently increases as the aneurysm grows. Abdominal aneurysms occur most commonly in Caucasian men between ages sixty and seventy. Individuals at high risk for aneurysms have high cholesterol levels, many years of heavy smoking, high blood pressure, and/or a family history of aneurysm.

Physical examination of the abdomen reveals a pulsating mass. X rays reveal the aneurysm if there is calcification in the vessel wall, and a CT scan is very good at identifying the extent and size of the lesions. Injecting intravenous dye to better determine the arteries included in the aneurysm is a procedure usually reserved for those who are candidates for surgery. Aneurysms of five centimeters or less can be watched, but those six centimeters or more require bypass surgery. This elective procedure is associated with 2 percent mortality, but the mortality rises to 30 percent once the vessel has ruptured.

DIABETIC NEUROPATHY

If glucose (sugar) levels get too high in the bloodstream of a diabetic for a long period of time, peripheral nerves that supply signals for sensation and muscle function are damaged. One of these nerves, the femoral, runs down the front of the thigh. Diabetes can cause a femoral neuropathy, which causes pain and weakness in the thigh.

Pain from peripheral neuropathy does not change with position, and this tells us it is not the kind of radicular pain we see with a disc herniation. The symptoms related to diabetes are improved when glucose levels return to normal, which is usually accomplished with oral medications or insulin injections.

An internist or endocrinologist can help you with the therapies necessary to control diabetes.

PAIN FROM NEARBY ORGANS

Abnormalities in organs that share nerves with part of the spine can cause referred back pain. It can arise from gastrointestinal, vascular, or genitourinary disorders. The duration and sequence of back pain follows the characteristics of the diseased organ. For example, colicky pain is characterized by repeated spasms of intense pain followed by pain-free periods. This kind of pain is associated with spasm in a hollow structure such as the ureter, colon, or gallbladder.

Anyone who has had a kidney stone understands severe colicky pain. Kidney and gall bladder pain occur in the upper portion of the lumbar spine while colonic pain occurs lower, near the sacrum. Abnormalities in these organ systems appear as blood in the urine or stool, or increasing pain when fatty foods are consumed. After eating spicy foods, individuals with ulcers in the stomach or small intestine may experience pain in the midline of the upper lumbar spine. It can often be quite difficult to determine the causes of the different types of back pain, and the job is made more difficult, of course, because the same person can experience pain from more than one cause.

Retroperitoneal Disorders

The retroperitoneum is the area in front of the lumbar spine. Any disorder that causes swelling in this area of the back causes pain that radiates from the low back through the front of the abdomen to the anterior thigh. The organs in the retroperitoneum include the kidneys, lymph glands, aorta, and large muscle groups (psoas). Kidney tumors, cancer of the lymph glands, aortic aneurysm, or bleeding into the large muscle groups can cause pain that appears in the anterior thigh, although its origin is in the lumbar spine. A MRI scan of the retroperitoneum will identify most of the organs that cause pain in this distribution.

BACK PAIN IN PREGNANCY AND MENSTRUATION

Half of all pregnant women develop moderate to severe back pain. This pain can be from hormonal changes that alter the flexibility of ligaments and joints in the pelvis, or simply the mechanical problem of the added weight in the pelvis. The pressure on the supporting structures in the pelvis or a marked increase in the lumbar curve (lordosis), strains the supporting muscles. In the nonpregnant state there is practically no motion in the joints of the pelvis, the front of the pelvis and sacroiliac joints. However, during pregnancy, a hormone, relaxin, is produced and it allows increased motion of the pelvic joints, and this causes tension in the relaxed capsule and ligaments. Increased lordosis also increases the weakness of the abdominal muscles and puts greater strain on the muscles near the spine. Active movement such as climbing stairs increases the strain.

Being physically fit before pregnancy may cut your risk of developing back pain. If a pregnancy is in your future, a physical fitness program with aerobic and strengthening exercises is helpful. If you are already pregnant and have back pain, exercises and external supports can be helpful to you.

You can decrease your back pain by lying on your side and by exercising in a swimming pool to strengthen your muscles while limiting strain on the lower extremities. Acetaminophen (Tylenol) is the only pain medication that is safe during pregnancy. In rare circumstances, if symptoms persist, a new mother may require bracing after delivery.

Most women find that extension exercises (bending backward) are most helpful (see chapter 8) The problem is that after the first three months, most moms are unable to rest on their stomachs to do this. You can do extension exercises while standing by placing your hands on the low back and bending backward. You can lean on a table and bend backward. Kneel on the floor and rest your upper body on a chair and increase the curve in your back.

If you have pain on one side of your back, try lying down on the side with the pain and put a small pillow at your waist.

Supporting your abdomen may also decrease pain. Place your hands under your abdomen and lift gently. If your back pain decreases, you are a candidate for a corset with a flexible band in front that expands as you enlarge through your pregnancy.

The good news is that back pain resolves when the baby is born. Only a very small minority of women continue to have pain months after the pregnancy is concluded.

Back pain that coincides with a woman's menstrual cycle may be related to endometriosis, a disease in which tissue from the lining of the uterus (endometrium) is present outside the uterine cavity. The endometrial tissue may be located on the ovaries or at the bottom of the pelvis near the rectum. Pain is a part of this disease because endometrial tissue outside the uterus undergoes the same monthly cycle of growth, shedding, and bleeding as the tissues inside the uterus. While the disease may occur at any age after the onset of menses, incidence rises as women reach their late twenties or thirties.

Overall, just over 3 percent of women of reproductive age develop endometriosis. When the endometriosis involves the colon and ureter, back pain is usually present. Pain increases at the time of menstruation and persists throughout the entire time of bleeding.

Endometriosis may render the abdomen tender over the uterus or ovary or other organs to which the endometrium has attached. Endometriosis is often diagnosed through laparoscopy, a relatively simple surgical procedure that allows us to view the inside of the abdomen. Organ tissue can be biopsied to determine the presence of endometrial tissue.

Endometriosis is usually treated with oral contraceptives or other medications that suppress menstruation, thereby suppressing the growth of the endometrium. Pregnancy will also suppress endometrial growth, but many women with endometriosis have difficulty conceiving because the disease leads to infertility.

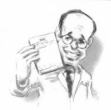

DR. B'S PRESCRIPTION SUMMARY

Rx

- "Red flags" are a sign of more serious systemic illness.

- Fever is associated with a back infection.

- Severe pain while lying down at night is caused by bone tumors.

- Prolonged morning stiffness is a characteristic of inflammatory arthritis of the spine.

- Bone pain is caused by fractures like those associated with osteoporosis.

- Crampy pain comes from other organs like the uterus, intestines, or ureter.

- Generalized muscle pain is caused by FM.

- TMS does not exist.

- Pregnant women can decrease back pain by exercising in a swimming pool to strengthen muscles while limiting strain on the legs, or by lying on their side.

Dr. B—

7

HOW AND WHEN TO USE MEDICATIONS EFFECTIVELY FOR PAIN

For the majority of those with back pain from mechanical disorders, a single drug is adequate to decrease pain. The more inflammatory the problem, the greater the need for a combination of multiple drug categories. Trial and error determine the best combination, and both patients and physicians can tire of this process, which unfortunately may lead to inadequate therapy. With some patients, I have tried *ten* different medications before finding the one that is effective and tolerated. I persisted because a drug regimen is so important in the prescription for low back pain. No single drug therapy is effective for all illnesses that cause spinal disease and pain. NSAIDs and analgesics have been proven effective for acute low back pain, but many back pain sufferers are resistant to using these medications even when the drugs make them feel better.

When I prescribed physical therapy and an NSAID to Chet, a forty-year-old carpenter, he refused the medication because he didn't want it to hide the pain and therefore lead to greater muscle damage. I explained to Chet that without relieving pain he would not be able to get the maximum benefit from his exercises. In his case, the prescription for his low back pain would be incomplete if he didn't agree to use the medications. If he performed his exercises with gradually increasing intensity and duration, the likelihood of causing extra muscle damage was small. Chet eventually relented and realized the NSAID allowed him to carry out his exercise program, and over the next month, his back pain disappeared. At that point he was able to stop taking the drug. As long as he continues his exercises, he can do his work. Chet is an example of the importance of looking at a back treatment prescription as an integrated whole, not just a group of options.

Many people are like Chet. They assume it's essential to feel pain in order to gauge improvement. This is simply not true. Drugs often effectively control pain while the underlying problem is improving. However, the medications do not always cure the underlying problem and once the medication is discontinued the pain may recur. Remember, too, that people with medical conditions that produce pain, such as arthritis, have used NSAIDs for decades without ill effects.

Even though NSAIDs and analgesics are not habit-forming narcotics, people may believe they are "addicted" to these medicines and dislike this sense of dependency. Mixed messages about drugs are all around us. On one hand, we hear the messages about illegal drugs and we are urged to work toward a "drug-free" society. On the other hand, we greatly value drugs with legitimate medical uses. How many lives would have been lost if antibiotics had not been developed? Sometimes patients confuse apples and oranges, and their concern about drugs in general adds to the stress associated with pain.

This fear of dependency is one reason people stop taking their pain medications too soon. Twenty-eight-year-old Lowell is a good example. He was in constant pain from a muscle strain caused by a skiing accident. This was aggravated when he twisted his spine, a motion his work required. In addition, not being able to ski for the two years since his accident both frustrated and depressed him. Exercises had not improved his condition.

Lowell was afraid of being becoming dependent on a drug in order to feel well, and he also was concerned about stomach irritation. I started him on Vioxx, a medication from one of the newer classes of drugs, the COX-2 inhibitor, and when it was clear that Lowell tolerated the drug, I increased his daily dose. In a short time his back pain resolved, along with full movement of his spine, and his blood tests were normal and showed no toxicity from his drug.

Two months later Lowell planned his first ski trip since his injury. However, his continued concern about his "drug dependency" led him to stop the medicine for a few days. Predictably, his pain returned. I reassured Lowell that even after taking the drug for four months, he was not "addicted" to Vioxx. He proved that to himself because he had stopped the medicine without any difficulty other than a return of his back pain. Furthermore, I could not tell him exactly how long he would need to take this medicine before his back pain resolved. I also emphasized that his ability to go on the ski trip was due to the effectiveness of the medication. After all, maximizing function is the primary goal of therapy. Taking a medication is the price we pay for function—and I believe it is a reasonable cost. Lowell took Vioxx during his trip and was able to enjoy skiing again.

NSAIDS AND COX-2 INHIBITORS

NSAIDs are nonsteroidal anti-inflammatory drugs, and they comprise the most frequently prescribed class of medicines. They are indicated for a variety of musculoskeletal diseases that affect the spine, including muscle injuries, herniated discs, osteoarthritis, and AS. NSAIDs reduce fever, pain, swelling, and clotting. These drugs are analgesic (painkillers) when taken in single doses. In larger doses over a longer period of time, they are also anti-inflammatory. Side effects include irritation to the stomach lining and—in very rare cases—stomach pain, holes in the intestinal wall, bowel blockage, and kidney failure.

Toxic side effects can be monitored with blood tests for liver and kidney function. The frequency of blood tests depends on your underlying health status. For example, young, healthy adults taking NSAIDs on a daily basis need blood tests once a year; older people with multiple medical problems may require monthly blood tests. While these NSAID-associated toxic effects are real, they are also manageable.

The new COX-2 inhibitors have eliminated many of these toxic side effects. Here's why: The production of hormone-like substances called prostaglandins (PGs) can be inhibited by an enzyme called cyclooxygenase (COX). Originally, a single COX enzyme was thought to regulate the production of PGs for the purpose of maintaining stomach lining and generating an inflammatory response. The NSAIDs decrease COX-1 activity, thus increasing the risk for stomach ulcers, leg swelling, and the bleeding associated with decreased platelet function. The degree to which normal functions are inhibited varies and is an individual response.

When a second COX enzyme was discovered, this advanced our understanding of the way NSAIDs work. COX-1 is present all the time and produces PGs that maintain organ function, including the stomach lining, blood pressure, and the airways in the lungs, and it helps maintain the correct balance of fluid in the body. COX-2 is an enzyme produced at sites of inflammation. The prostaglandins produced by COX-2 are associated with heat and swelling and redness and pain in affected areas. When we inhibit COX-2 we can control inflammation and pain to about the same degree as occurred with the older NSAIDs, but with less toxicity. So the new COX-2 inhibitors are "safer aspirin," not "super aspirin."

Finding the Right NSAID for Your Pain

NSAIDs and COX-2 inhibitors currently available for the treatment of spinal disorders are listed in appendix B. The choice and dosage of NSAIDs depend on factors related to your medical condition. Acute mechanical conditions (muscle strain) occurring in young people require NSAIDs with rapid onset of action and pain-relieving properties, such as ibuprofen, naproxen, ketoprofen, rofecoxib. For these acute mechanical disorders, treatment with NSAIDs generally lasts two to four weeks. Concerns about toxicity are less significant if, for example, you are young with a muscle strain that will improve in a short period and you do not have any other medical problem.

NSAIDs available over the counter include ibuprofen (Advil, Motrin Ib, Nuprin), naproxen (Aleve), and ketoprofen (Orudis KT). These same drugs are available in prescription strength: Motrin, Naprelan, and Orudis, respectively. If the OTC products are taken in high doses, they will have the same benefits and toxicities as their prescription counterparts. These over-the-counter medications have a lower, but continued, risk of toxicity. Since most adults routinely take these products for minor pain, the best advice I can give you is to follow the instructions on the pill container, but if your symptoms do not subside, see your doctor. Do not take more without your doctor's advice.

Aspirin, a powerful NSAID, improves low back pain and is effective but potentially toxic. The same properties that make aspirin effective for preventing heart attacks and strokes also increase the risk for bleeding. In addition to stomach ulcers, aspirin can cause ringing in the ears, reversible deafness, and death if taken in a high dosage. Never exceed the recommended dose without advice from your doctor.

Use a COX-2 inhibitor if you have a history of stomach ulcer. If you are taking either an NSAID or COX-2 inhibitor on a daily basis, you should have your weight and blood pressure measured regularly. Some NSAIDs can increase fluid retention and blood pressure, and blood tests also are indicated to monitor for toxicities affecting blood counts and kidney and liver function.

Understanding Timing and Dosage

Dosages of NSAIDs and COX-2 inhibitors vary based on the length of time they stay in your body. This is known as the drug's half-life. For example, NSAIDs that are eliminated from the body more slowly require fewer pills per day for a sustained anti-inflammatory effect. NSAIDs and COX-2 inhibitors with long half-lives include piroxicam, oxaprozin, rofecoxib, celecoxib, and meloxicam. Some NSAIDs are eliminated rapidly but can be given once or twice a day in sustained release formulations. Examples include naproxen, ketoprofen, etodolac, indomethacin, and diclofenac.

If a medication helps for a portion of the day but then loses effect, an additional dose at the end of a day may be appropriate. If a drug is somewhat toxic, it may be easier on you if you limit your intake of alcohol and coffee. Smoking can also exacerbate drug toxicities. If NSAIDs are not effective, and if you have a history of stomach ulcers or if you take corticosteroids, you are an appropriate candidate for COX-2 inhibitors.

NSAIDs and COX-2 inhibitors come in different sizes and forms, including tablets, capsules, and liquids. The pills may be small or large. All these factors may play a role in deciding which is the best drug for you. For example, Celecoxib comes in 100 mg and 200 mg tablets. The dosage for an older person with osteoarthritis might be 200 mg, while someone with severe pain might be taking 800 mg a day. Celecoxib has greatest activity in the body over an eleven-hour period and is usually prescribed twice a day. However, for many people, a 200 mg tablet once a day is adequate to control the symptoms of arthritis.

Vioxx comes in tablets of various strengths and is also available in liquid form. It is active in the body for eighteen hours and needs to be taken once a day. Some older people do well with 12.5 mg once a day; others with more acutely painful problems require 50 mg a day. Some people prefer to decide if they need extra medicine on a particular day. They will take 25 mg in the morning, and if they are experiencing more pain, they will take an additional 25 mg.

The future holds great promise for more effective and safer COX-2 inhibitors, and the second generation of COX-2 inhibitors is currently being studied in clinical trials. These medicines may offer more anti-inflammatory effects with less toxicity than currently available COX-2 inhibitors. The results of the clinical trials will define their benefits and guide us as we determine their future role in pain management.

NSAIDs should be taken with food to decrease stomach toxicities, but COX-2 inhibitors can be taken on an empty stomach. You should review the doses of all your medications, and how you take them, with your physician.

MUSCLE RELAXANTS

The Agency for Health Care Policy and Research (AHCPR) has reviewed studies of muscle relaxants and concluded that they are probably as helpful as NSAIDs for low back pain, but they cause drowsiness in 30 percent of those taking them and are prescribed infrequently.

I have found that muscle relaxants are particularly helpful for muscle strain and its associated spasm. A recent study from a health maintenance organization in the state of Washington reported that an NSAID and a muscle relaxant were the most effective combination of medications for people with acute low back pain. Muscle relaxants can also be effective for chronic low back pain when you have limited motion because of muscle tightness.

The combination of NSAIDs and muscle relaxants is effective for reversing the "pain-spasm cycle," characterized by muscle pain that causes increasing muscle spasm, and, thus, more pain and more spasm. An analgesic and muscle relaxant allows treatment of both components of the cycle. Treating just one component of the cycle may not correct the problem because either the pain or the spasm persists. A complete prescription requires both classes of drugs if you have muscle spasm.

We still do not know exactly how muscle relaxants work, but we do know they do not work directly on the muscles in the arms and legs. Their effect is on the central nervous system, which controls the tension in muscles. Thus, they work to reverse tension in the damaged muscle.

Like NSAIDs, beneficial response to muscle relaxants varies with the individual and so trial and error is sometimes necessary. I usually start patients on the lowest dose, taken two hours before sleep. Since the action of most muscle relaxants is delayed, taking them in the evening before sleep eliminates problems created by drowsiness. Muscle relaxants currently available are listed in appendix B.

Lucy's back pain had a detrimental effect on her work as computer programmer, but also made it difficult to take care of her twelve-year-old child. She had so much difficulty walking that her twelve-year-old daughter was helping her put on her clothes and doing all the household chores. Lucy was becoming increasingly concerned about the burden her daughter was carrying. She was supposed to be practicing the violin, not taking care of her mother.

Examination revealed a severe degree of muscle spasm in the right buttock and lower back muscles. Although she had received NSAIDs in the past, she had never been given a muscle relaxant. I prescribed cyclobenzaprine (Flexeril), three times a day, along with her naproxen. Within two weeks, her back pain had decreased, and although she was still stiff, she was able to pick up more of the household chores. Lucy also started a stretching exercise program, and within another month she returned to work. Drug doses decreased over the next year, and she eventually used exercises exclusively as the means to control her pain and was able to sit comfortably at her daughter's violin recital.

A wide range of muscle relaxants is available. Some of the medications include cyclobenzaprine (Flexeril), orphenadrine (Norflex), chlorzoxazone (Parafon Forte), and metaxalone (Skelaxin). I do not use the muscle relaxant diazepam (Valium) because, unlike other muscle relaxants, it has a tendency to cause depression when used for a long time. These drugs are used while increased muscle spasm and decreased range of motion are present and quickly withdrawn once muscle spasm is resolved.

NARCOTIC AND NON-NARCOTIC ANALGESICS

If you are unable to tolerate NSAIDs, you may benefit from analgesics. The pure analgesics reduce pain but have no effect on a disease's inflammatory component and, therefore, are not preferred therapy in many circumstances. Pain-relieving medications—analgesics—are divided into nonnarcotic and narcotic groups.

Nonnarcotic Analgesics

Acetaminophen (Tylenol) is a pure analgesic without any anti-inflammatory effects. It works by decreasing PG production in the central nervous system but has no effect on the production of PG in the rest of the body. Acetaminophen is a less-effective analgesic than aspirin, but it has none of the toxic side effects such as stomach ulcers or breathing difficulties associated with the NSAIDs. If you have aspirin sensitivity, acetaminophen should be the first pain therapy you take. It should also be considered if you are older and have osteoarthritis of the spine. It can be used in combination with NSAIDs or narcotic drugs.

Check with your physician to determine the maximum dose of acetaminophen that is appropriate for your clinical condition. Be especially cautious if you drink alcohol on a daily basis and take acetaminophen, because both drugs irritate the liver. If you drink alcohol regularly, you must lower your dose of the drug. In order to decrease the risk of liver damage while on high doses of acetaminophen, you will need blood tests that monitor liver function.

Acetaminophen is available in a variety of doses (325 mg, 500 mg, 650 mg) and forms (tablets, capsules, liquid). Tylenol Arthritis is special in that the effect of the medicine is prolonged. Where the effect of regular acetaminophen is about four hours, Tylenol Arthritis is released more slowly and has a six- to eight-hour effect. Taken three times a day, this drug is able to offer pain relief around the clock.

Tramadol (Ultram) is another nonnarcotic, pure analgesic that is as effective as aspirin and ibuprofen. Its action is mediated through activation of narcotic and serotonin receptors in the central nervous system. Like acetaminophen, tramadol has no cross-reaction with NSAIDs, and if you are sensitive to aspirin you can take tramadol without concern about difficulty breathing. This drug also has no effect on stomach lining, although tramadol may cause nausea and dizziness. Do not take tramadol if you have a history of seizures, because it lowers seizure threshold, thereby increasing the risk of seizure occurance.

Tramadol comes as a 50 mg tablet that can be broken into 25 mg halves. You should start the drug at 25 mg to decrease the risk of nausea. You can increase the dose as tolerated after consultation with your physician. Most people benefit at less than the maximum dose. Like acetaminophen, tramadol is synergistic and can be used with NSAIDs for additional pain relief.

Narcotic Analgesics

We do not need narcotic analgesics such as codeine, hydrocodone, meperidine, morphine, or fentanyl to treat acute low back pain. However, if you have severe sciatica related to a herniated disc, narcotic analgesics, used along with NSAIDS and muscle relaxants, are part of your complete prescription to ease pain. The risk of developing dependency is the major toxicity of narcotics, so they are stopped as soon as possible. Narcotic drugs attach to the receptors in the pain-reducing pathway in the central nervous system.

Narcotic analgesics are of limited use for treating chronic low back pain. In the past, narcotics needed to be given every few hours because their analgesic effects wore off quickly. Recently, narcotic drugs with prolonged action have been developed, including Oxycontin, Kadian, MS Contin, and Durgagesic. These drugs can be dosed orally twice a day or in patch form once every three days.

These narcotic analgesics improve physical function of chronic pain patients with failed back surgery (see chapter 10) and those with direct nerve damage associated with persistent sciatica. The dose of drug is increased until pain is controlled. Increasing the dose beyond this level of pain control does not increase the efficacy of the drug, but it does increase the risk of toxicity. In addition to dependency, narcotics cause constipation and sleepiness.

Fortunately, relatively few people require chronic narcotic therapy, but for those individuals, these drugs are essential for a functional quality of life. Both you and your physician should be comfortable with the choice before committing to chronic, long-acting narcotic therapy.

You and your physician must review the benefits and detriments of these drugs before you start taking them. While narcotics do not always make people "high," some of these drugs depress mood, and they can cause headaches, disorientation, and constipation.

For home use, the narcotic of choice is codeine. Other narcotics, such as oxycodone or hydrocodone, in varying combinations with aspirin or acetaminophen, are also useful to decrease pain in the appropriate individuals. The goal is to decrease the use of these medications as soon as pain is decreased.

CORTICOSTEROIDS

Glucocorticoids, such as prednisone, are not related to androgenic steroids that athletes take to build muscles, and they are not toxic. Your body actually makes the equivalent of 7.5 mg of prednisone every day. The difference is that the body-made corticosteroids are released all day long whereas the pharmaceutical prednisone is absorbed all at one time.

Some people fear steroid medication because they have heard that common side effects are increased appetite and weight gain, but this does not happen to everyone. Other side effects include high blood pressure, cataracts, diabetes, and osteoporosis, but these problems come with long-term use. Always discuss side effects with your physician, because once recognized, they can be treated.

Oral corticosteroids are reserved for people with severe pain or muscle weakness that has not improved with NSAIDs alone. The decision to use corticosteroids should be made after your entire medical condition is reviewed. I prefer to order low doses of prednisone for an extended period of time. Other physicians prefer a larger dose of corticosteroids, which is then tapered over a seven-day course. Low doses for a short period of time reduce potential toxic side effects. Once improvement is achieved, the steroids are tapered. If no improvement occurs at four weeks, the steroids are quickly discontinued.

In rare circumstances, a low dose of prednisone may be used to treat spinal stenosis. Patients who are resistant to epidural injections (see following discussion), have had maximum NSAID therapy, and have refused decompression surgery generally remain incapacitated, even unable to walk short distances. In these very specialized circumstances, low-dose prednisone may be helpful.

Response to the drug needs to be constantly monitored. If signs of improvement disappear, the medicine should be discontinued.

Epidural Corticosteroid Injection Therapy

Oral corticosteroids are easy to take, but the disadvantage is they are systemic and affect your entire body. Epidural corticosteroid injections are safe, and complications, infections, or toxicities are rare. Improvement does not occur immediately, and the corticosteroids need days to decrease nerve swelling. Up to a week may be needed before you notice an improvement in leg pain, but improvement lasts for months. Epidural injections should be considered if you do not respond to oral drug therapy and are reluctant to undergo lumbar spine surgery.

The epidural space is inside the spinal canal but outside the covering of the spinal cord (dura). Herniated disc and spinal stenosis compression occur near the epidural space. Epidural corticosteroids have a greater anti-inflammatory effect because the medication comes in direct contract with the inflamed nerve root. The injection is given at the base of the spine near the coccyx (tailbone), or in the lumbar area. The success of the injection can depend on the experience of the health care professional placing the needle. Anesthesiologists have extensive experience with epidural injections.

No study has determined the correct number of epidural injections to achieve the maximum effect, but the number should be kept to the minimum. If one injection is adequate for symptom relief, additional injections are not indicated. Epidural injections are limited to a set of three every six months, since no additional benefit is noted with more injections. Injections are given no more frequently than every two weeks with the set of three completed over six to eight weeks. People with spinal stenosis can have injections repeated every six months.

One of the misconceptions about epidural corticosteroid injections involves the rapidity of improvement. Some people are disappointed when they do not see immediate reduction in discomfort from sciatica. However, corticosteroids work more slowly than anesthetics. These steroids work by decreasing the inflammation of the disc and nerve, a process that takes time.

Iontophoresis: Another Form of "Injection" Therapy

Iontophoresis is a machine that uses direct electrical current from a 9-volt battery to transfer a medicine across a body surface without the need for an injection. Local anesthetics and soluble corticosteroids are the medicines most frequently given by iontophoresis. The medicine is injected into a pad that is placed over the painful area. The treatment takes about twenty minutes to complete. The frequency of treatments corresponds to the pain relief. The treatment cannot be repeated too frequently because of the buildup of corticosteroids. However, treatments can be given intermittently, over extended periods of time. On occasion, iontophoresis delivers local pain relief that can have significant effects on overall function.

A fifty-eight-year-old man's hobby was riding motorcycles. Over the past two years, his riding had decreased because he would experience right buttock pain that would increase over time. He had tried medicines but had an NSAID sensitivity that prevented his use of NSAIDs and COX-2 medications. He had tried local injections in the past but had none recently. He had developed atrial fibrillation, a fluttering of the heart that required taking blood thinners on a daily basis. He would bleed excessively with any injections. He was depressed because he could not get back out on his bike. My suggestion was that he try iontophoresis over his painful buttock area. The therapy was helpful, and pain relief lasted for an extended period of time. He used the therapy intermittently when he had a return of pain and he was going to ride his motorcycle.

Iontophoresis can be used for pain in other superficial locations. This therapy is applied by physical therapists with a prescription from a physician for the therapy and the medication. Some physicians also offer the therapy in their offices.

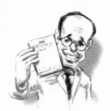

DR. B'S PRESCRIPTION SUMMARY

℞

- Anti-inflammatory drug therapy decreases pain and inflammation and helps keep you functioning.

- Muscle relaxants decrease muscle spasms when used in combination with NSAIDs.

- Analgesics—both non-narcotic and narcotic—relieve pain but do not decrease inflammation

- Maximizing the beneficial effects of drug therapy is a trial and error process. You may need to try a few different kinds of medications to find the most pain relief with the fewest side effects.

- Spinal injections with corticosteroids are helpful in resolving sciatica secondary to a herniated disc. Steroids can be delivered through the skin without a needle with electrical current from a battery (iontophoresis).

Dr. B—

8

TREATMENT WITH EXERCISE AND PHYSICAL THERAPY

Exercise and physical therapy can be very important to the treatment of low back pain as long as you know when to use them. Exercise can increase motion and improve healing to an area that has been injured. A physical therapist can recommend exercises and similar therapies to improve and maintain the function of your lumbar spine.

A wide range of exercises is available for the treatment and prevention of low back pain. Flexion (bending forward) and extension (bending backward) are the most widely recommended. Choosing the appropriate exercise program is important, because the wrong exercises can make things worse. You may feel comfortable deciding for yourself, or you could be evaluated by a physical therapist.

WORKING WITH A PHYSICAL THERAPIST

Physical therapy is useful for low back pain if given at the appropriate time. If given too early, you are too "hot"—meaning that pain is so acute that any attempt to improve movement causes increased muscle spasm resulting in

107

marked pain. Exercise can make acute back pain worse if you begin too early in the course of recovery from a back injury, according to a study by the Agency for Health Care Policy and Research (AHCPR), an organization that published therapy guidelines in 1994. Stretching back muscles or doing strength exercises in the early stages of an episode of acute low back pain can cause greater pain.

The time for exercises is when pain starts to decrease and movement is increasing. You can start with simple flexion and extension exercises without a visit to a physical therapist, but if back pain is not going away and you still can't move any better, then a physical therapist can be helpful to improve function. There are many reasons for completing a course of physical therapy and exercise:

- To decrease the pain
- To strengthen your muscles
- To stretch your muscles
- To decrease stress to your spinal structures
- To improve fitness to reduce chance of recurrence
- To stabilize your back problem
- To improve your posture
- To improve your mobility

As we age, intervertebral discs are pancakes, not pillows. Therefore, the discs are unable to sustain as many shocks. We must consider new ways to use our back muscles and body position to protect our spine. Physical therapy and exercises help us reach that goal.

No single set of exercise works for all causes of acute and chronic low back pain. In independent studies, flexion and extension exercises are shown to be helpful for chronic low back pain. In a study examining both flexion and extension exercises in the same group of people with low back pain, both sets of exercises were helpful, with flexion exercises resulting in significantly improved front-to-back motion. Before you begin any of these exercises, check with your doctor or health care provider to be sure they are appropriate for you.

One more precaution. Many of my patients have confused the role of a physical trainer with that of a physical therapist. Physical trainers have expertise in exercises to maximize function. The role of these trainers is that of drill sergeant to maximize your exercise to the point of exhaustion. These exercises may be indicated when you are well, but they may put you at risk if your back has not fully healed. A physical therapist works with people who are unable to function in their daily activities because of physical pain. Do not confuse them.

FLEXION EXERCISES

The mechanism by which exercises produce pain relief is not completely known, but many reasons make common sense. Back and leg pain can come from compression of nerves when enlarged facet joints narrow the neural foramen. Bending forward would open these holes for the nerves and decrease nerve compression. Flexion stretches tight muscles that move the hip and low back in a backward direction and strengthens abdominal and buttock muscles. In addition, increasing intra-abdominal pressure has the potential of increased support of the lumbar spine. Do not use flexion exercises if you have a herniated disc or if you have leg pain in a seated position. Do use flexion exercises if you have:

- Pain in the low back with prolonged standing and relief when you sit

- Pain in the low back when you bend backward and relief when you bend forward

- Spondylolisthesis (the front of your spinal column is not attached to the back of the column)

- Spinal stenosis (leg pain with walking that is relieved with sitting)

Do flexion exercises in the proper sequence—from a resting state to stretching and then to stretching and strengthening. You can use an exercise table or a mat on the floor. Never do flexion exercises with both legs straight. This increases tension in the psoas muscle, in front of the lumbar spine. Increased tension in this muscle increases the pressure in the spinal discs and may increase pain in your back. In fact, doing sit-ups this way can give you a back pain if you don't already have one.

Acute Relaxation Phase

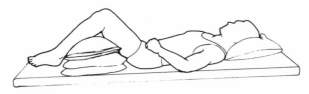

Figure 8.1 Resting position. Flex your hips with pillows under your knees for fifteen minutes.

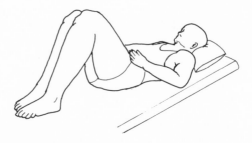

Figure 8.2 Resting position. Do it without pillows for fifteen minutes.

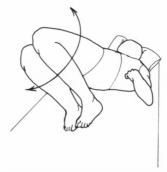

Figure 8.3 Back rotation. Keep your shoulders on the table or floor while you turn your pelvis and legs with your knees together. Turn to one side as much as you can tolerate or for one minute. Alternate sides.

Stretching Phase

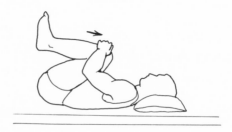

Figure 8.4 Pull your knees up to your chest while raising your pelvis. Hold this for a count of three and relax to the count of six. Begin with one leg at a time and advance to both legs as you improve.

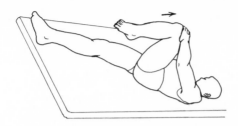

Figure 8.5 Crossover leg exercise. Place your heel on your opposite knee and pull the bent knee across your body to the opposite shoulder. Hold for a count of three and then relax for the count of six. Alternate legs and do 10 repetitions.

Stretching and Strengthening Phase

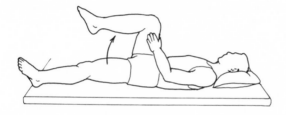

Figure 8.6 Hamstring stretch with knee bent. Bend your knee and flex your hip for a count of three and then relax for a count of six.

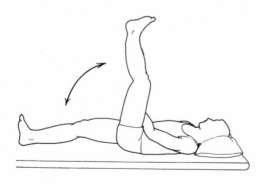

Figure 8.7 Hamstring stretch with straight leg. Hold for three, then relax for six.

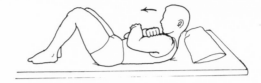

Figure 8.8 Partial sit up. Bend your knees and put your arms on your chest. Hold for three then relax for a count of six. Repeat this with variation from the easiest to most difficult: arms straight out, arms folded on chest, hands behind head.

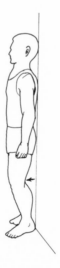

Figure 8.9 Pelvic tilt in standing position. Every hour flatten your low back against a wall with your knees bent. Hold for a count of three every hour. This movement is not only basic to sexual intercourse but is also one of the best ways to stretch the muscles on the back of the spine and strengthen the front ones. The pelvic tilt can be done with a small, nonprovocative motion even in the presence of others. This exercise can be done when sitting, standing, or lying flat. Try it, you'll like it.

Isometric Back Flexion Exercises

Paul Williams's flexion exercises use motion to improve muscle function as illustrated in figures 8.6 through 8.9. Another form of flexion exercises improves muscle function without any movement. These are isometric exercises—meaning that the muscle contracts but does not move. Use these exercises if even small motions of your back cause pain. Isometrics can strengthen muscles but do not promote flexibility.

Start isometric back flexion exercises by pushing down on your abdominal muscles as if you were forcing a bowel movement. This is the Valsalva maneuver. The same process that works with that bodily function contracts muscles in the abdomen. As you close off your throat and push, your abdominal muscles contract but do not move. Count from five to fifteen as you can tolerate it, then rest. Work up to sets of ten to fifteen repetitions three to four times a day.

The next set of exercises involves the buttocks. Squeeze your cheeks (the gluteus muscles) together. Count between five to fifteen, then rest. If you are coordinated, try a Valsalva maneuver and cheek squeeze together. The result of these two actions is a sustained pelvic tilt with tightened buttock muscles. These exercises strengthen the flexor muscles and give you greater stability.

EXTENSION EXERCISES

In contrast to Paul Williams flexion exercises, Robin McKenzie, a physical therapist from New Zealand, proposed extension exercises as a means to decrease pain. He suggested that leg pain came from a disc herniation pressing on a spinal nerve and by bending backward you could force the ruptured part of the disc back to its normal location. However, this method has not proven effective in relieving sciatica. Nerve compression causes leg numbness, not pain. Nerve inflammation causes sciatic pain. (Neither Williams's nor McKenzie's exercise methods acutely changes inflammation in an irritated spinal nerve.)

The purpose of extension exercises is to strengthen the muscles along the spine and to improve your endurance and spinal mobility, and also to increase the stamina of the lumbar spine, center the gel—or cushion—inside the disc, and decrease your risk of reinjury. Do extension exercises if you have:

- Pain in the low back with prolonged sitting or driving
- Pain in the low back with bending forward
- Pain in the low back rising from a chair

113

- Pain in the leg that is increased with sitting
- Relief with lying flat
- Relief with walking

Extension exercises should follow a progression during the early phase of low back pain:

Acute Relaxation Phase

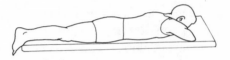

Figure 8.10 Lie facedown with pillows under your abdomen. Add more pillows as you can tolerate it. Do this for fifteen minutes.

Stretching Phase

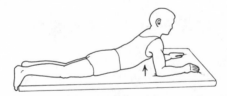

Figure 8.11 Prop yourself up on bent elbows and hold for three then relax to count of six.

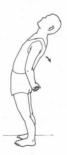

Figure 8.12 Place your hands on your low back and bend backwards. Hold for three then relax to count of six. Repeat this hourly.

Treatment with Exercise and Physical Therapy

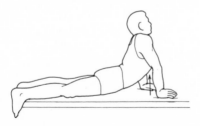

Figure 8.13 Prop yourself up on outstretched arms (like a push up movement). Hold for ten and do ten repetitions.

Strengthening Phase

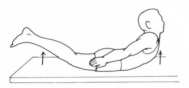

Figure 8.14 Raise your head and legs off the floor as much as you can tolerate. Hold this position for a count of three and then relax to a count of six.

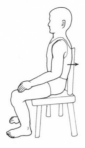

Figure 8.15 Now raise yourself up and maintain a normal seated posture with curved back.

Variations

A variation to extension strengthening exercises can be tried when you are "on all fours." Attempt this only after your back pain has begun to improve. Stretch out your arm and the opposite leg parallel to the floor. Hold this position for a count of two and then return your arm and leg to the floor. Do the same motion with the opposite arm and leg. Try to increase repetitions in the "Comfort Zone" as you tolerate. You should try for a goal of ten to fifteen lifts.

After two weeks of doing these flexion and extension exercises, you can add another set of exercises to your routine:

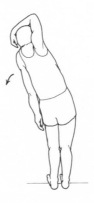

Figure 8.16 Lateral bending in the standing position. Put your hand on opposite side of your head with the other arm sliding down your leg. Hold for a count of ten and repeat every hour.

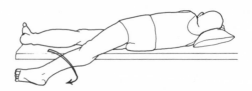

Figure 8.17 Lying on your side. Hold your top leg straight and move it behind you. Hold for three then relax for six.

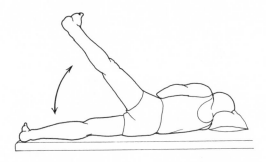

Figure 8.18 Lying on your side, raise your leg away from your body. Hold for three then relax for six.

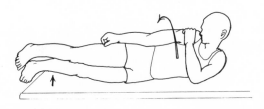

Figure 8.19 Lying on your side, lift your head and legs off the bed. Hold for three then relax for six.

THE "C" AND "S" CURVES

Sometimes muscles are in so much spasm that the spine is bent into a "C" or an "S." Not everyone has spasm to this degree, but there's something that can help you find out if you do. An experienced physical therapist, Tom Welsh, taught me that people could determine the exercises that would help their back curve. Here are his suggestions. First, decide which letter of the alphabet, "C" or "S," best fits your shape. Stand in front of a full-length mirror and compare the height of your shoulders and hips.

Use your right and left arms or legs depending on the type of curve you have. Do these on the floor or in bed. These exercises improve flexibility but also stabilize the spine, which improves function and decreases pain.

RIGHT "C" CURVE

LEFT "C" CURVE

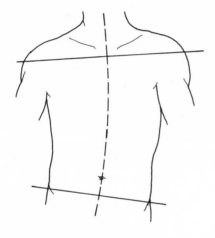

Figure 8.20 Right "C"—the left shoulder and right hip are higher

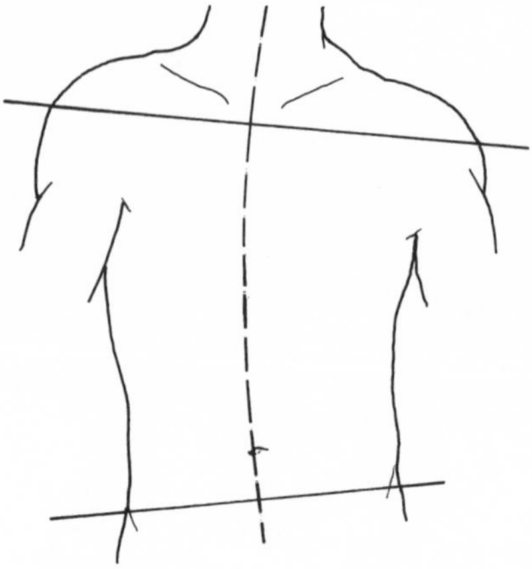

Figure 8.21 Left "C"—the right shoulder and left hip are higher

FRONT "S" CURVE

BACKWARD "S" CURVE

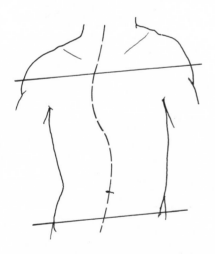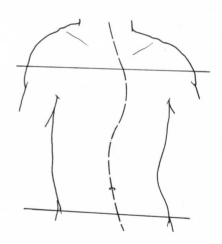

Figure 8.22 Front "S"—the left shoulder and left hip are higher

Figure 8.23 Backward "S"—the right shoulder and right hip are higher

Treatment with Exercise and Physical Therapy

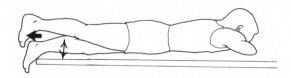

Figure 8. 24 Exercise 1—Lie on Your Stomach. Raise a straight leg a few inches off the bed and overstretch it downward. Hold for a count of three. Repeat ten times. (Right "C" and Front "S"—left leg; Left "C" and Backward "S"—right leg.)

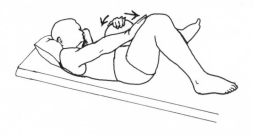

Figure 8.25 Exercise 2—Lie on your back. Bend your knees. Raise a bent knee and push your hand against the knee with equal resistance. At the same time pull your opposite knee towards your chest. Hold for a count of three. Repeat ten times. (Right "C" and Front "S"—raise right knee and pull left knee; Left "C" and Backward "S"—raise left knee and pull right knee.)

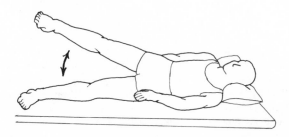

Figure 8.26 Exercise 3—Lie on your side. Align your legs with your body. Raise the top leg up and down twelve to eighteen inches. Repeat twenty-five times. (Right "C" and Front "S"—left side down, right leg raises; Left "C" and Backward "S"—right side down, left leg raises.)

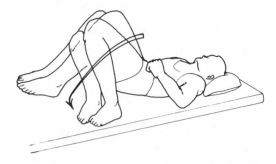

Figure 8.27 Exercise 4—Lie on your back. Bend your knees and keep your knees and heels together. Roll both knees to the side. Hold for a count of twenty. Tighten your stomach muscles and keep them tight while you roll your knees back to the center. Repeat three times. (Right "C"—roll right; Left "C"—roll left.)

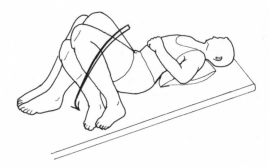

Figure 8.28 Exercise 5—Lie on your back. Bend your knees and keep your knees and heels together. Put a pillow under your shoulder and upper back. Roll both knees to the side with the pillow. Hold for a count of twenty. Tighten your stomach muscles and keep them tight while you roll your knees back to the center. Repeat three times. (Front "S"—pillow left shoulder, roll left; Backward "S"—pillow right shoulder, roll right.)

Treatment with Exercise and Physical Therapy

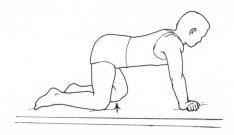

Figure 8.29 Exercise 6—Get down on your hands and knees. Align your knees with your hips and your hands with your shoulders. Raise your knee up and down one to two inches. Repeat twenty-five times. (Right "C" and Backward "S"—raise left knee; Left "C" and Front "S"—raise right knee.)

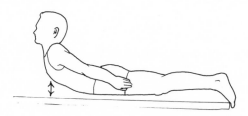

Figure 8.30 Exercise 7—Lie on your stomach. Keep your arms at your sides. Raise your chest and shoulders up and down and arch your back. Repeat this twenty-five times at a rapid pace. (All curves.)

TRANSCUTANEOUS ELECTRICAL NERVE STIMULATION (TENS)

Physical therapists sometimes use TENS therapy with surface electrodes applied to the skin. (Electrodes can be implanted directly on a nerve or sensory column of the spinal cord, but only by a neurosurgeon.)

TENS works by stimulating high-speed nerve fibers that block the slower speed pain fibers. Different forms of electrical signals are needed to stimulate nerve fibers. The settings on the TENS machine (transcutaneous stimulator) are modified to find the correct wave pulse that works best for you.

Once the appropriate setting is reached, you will feel a tingling sensation

121

in the stimulated area. The sensation should not cause an unpleasant sensation or muscle contracture. Therapy sessions should last for a minimum of thirty minutes to determine if therapy has benefit. The onset of pain relief can be measured from minutes to hours. The average time is twenty minutes. The duration of pain relief is variable. Some people have had relief lasting days to weeks from a short course of therapy. TENS does not work for everyone.

. . .

Exercises are only as good as the frequency with which they are done. I have given many printed and illustrated exercise directions to patients who promise that they will do their exercises religiously. They return a bit sheepish admitting that they had no time in their schedules for what they knew would be helpful to their condition.

The best successes I have had are with people who followed their exercise routine on a regular basis. They stopped their medicines and remained functional even though at times the beneficial response was delayed. For example, a forty-eight-year-old cabinetmaker developed back pain after standing in an extended posture for a number of hours while installing a set of heavy cabinets. He developed severe muscle spasm and increased back pain with extending his spine. I gave him an NSAID and a muscle relaxant for relief of his symptoms. Then I educated him about the importance of flexion exercises and the danger of bending backwards. He gradually improved, and within one month he was back at work building and installing cabinets. He could not stop his medicines without developing a return of his back pain. He wanted to stop his medicines but had to continue to work. I told him to continue to do his exercises on a regular basis. He did his exercises religiously. After a year, he did not need his muscle relaxant. He was about ready to stop his NSAID when he stopped exercising. He had a relapse of his pain. He returned to his exercises and within the next year was able to stop all his medicine. Currently, he is building cabinets, doing his exercises, and staying off medicines.

Exercises do make a difference. A flexible and strong lower back is an anchor to a number of our daily activities. If you put in the work, you will gain the benefit.

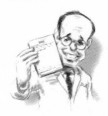

DR. B'S PRESCRIPTION SUMMARY

R~

- Exercises and physical therapy play a greater role during the later healing phase of healing acute low back pain.

- No one type of exercise program fits all types of back pain, but flexion (bending forward) and extension (bending backward) exercises are most widely recommended by doctors and physical therapists.

- Exercises are also important if you have chronic low back pain because they will stretch and strengthen your back muscles and help improve mobility and reduce pain.

- Exercises are most effective when you do them regularly.

- A physical trainer is not the same as a physical therapist.

Dr. B—

9

COMPLEMENTARY THERAPIES

Cultures throughout the world have used healing techniques that today fall into the category of complementary therapy. Some of these therapies were accepted in India and China, for example, well before scientific methods became available to prove their effectiveness for improving certain medical conditions. We still do not know the mechanism of action for some complementary therapies, and some physicians and others believe the benefits are largely a placebo effect. But whatever the effect, more attention is being paid in medical schools and by practicing physicians. For instance, some conventional doctors have actually learned how to give acupuncture treatments.

In 1997 an estimated 629 million visits were made to practitioners of complementary therapies, while only 388 million were made to primary care physicians. Four of ten Americans use complementary therapies to some extent. Low back pain sufferers are frequent visitors to practitioners of complementary medicine such as chiropractors, acupuncturists, and bodywork specialists. Complementary therapies seem most popular among those who cannot find satisfaction with conventional therapies, or who have a condition that is unpredictable—such as low back pain. Such therapies are also considered relatively risk free and cheaper than conventional medicine. Without choosing well, however, none of these considerations are true.

The term "complementary medicine" implies that such therapies are used in concert with conventional therapies for low back pain, while the term "alternative" therapy suggests that these therapies are mutually exclusive, which is not the case. However, I view complementary methods as passive therapies, which, for the most part, are done *to* back pain patients. This is particularly true of chiropractic, osteopathic, and bodywork therapies. I prefer active therapies such as education about self-directed exercise regimens that enable you to take control of your condition.

You may seek complementary therapies based on a friend's recommendation, an advertisement, or past experience. Regardless of the reason, tell your doctor about every vitamin, natural supplement, special diet, exercise, or manual therapy you are using. Your physician may have experience with complementary practitioners and, therefore, offer recommendations.

These therapies are here to stay. Some can help your back pain, but use them wisely and only to:

• Enhance the effects of conventional therapies
• Improve your outlook
• Ease symptoms of chronic pain, stress, and anxiety

In general, complementary therapies *cannot:*

• Cure any illness
• Improve acute illnesses rapidly
• Replace conventional therapies

MANUAL MANIPULATION

A prominent group of complementary therapists, including chiropractors, osteopaths, and massage therapists, believe that the natural healing processes of the body are facilitated through manipulation and movement of soft tissues and repositioning of body parts. They believe their treatments remove blockages and result in improved function by moving the spine back to its normal position. Some disciplines believe that a variety of illnesses can be treated through this manipulation of the musculoskeletal system, but this remains controversial.

Chiropractic Manipulation

Chiropractic manipulation seems to be most effective for acute low back pain of short duration, usually a month or less. Some people improve with the first session; others require several treatments. If a month of therapy has passed without improvement, chiropractic treatment will not help you.

Studies show the benefit of chiropractic manipulation for low back pain without sciatica, but these benefits are short term, and chronic low back pain does not appear to benefit from chiropractic therapy. Occasionally, chiropractic adjustment may encourage movement in those with limited motion and chronic back pain.

In certain situations, manipulation can have serious effects on your health. For example, it is not recommended for people with sciatica (leg pain). Adjustments may make a disc herniation worse, causing loss of strength or loss of bladder and rectal function.

Older people should be especially cautious about chiropractic adjustment if they have osteoporosis or small fractures in a vertebra. There is added risk if you are taking blood-thinning medication. Some of the chiropractic adjustments can cause bleeding. If you have one of these conditions, consult with a medical doctor before undergoing chiropractic manipulation because the treatment may not be safe for you.

The premise of chiropractic therapy is that misaligned vertebrae (subluxations) cause most illness by blocking the nervous system and interfering with natural healing. Adjusting the spine to its natural position reverses this process, resulting in a cure. Chiropractors make adjustments with gentle pressures or more forceful thrusts to the spine. Sometimes this generates a popping sound like cracking knuckles, which is actually a bubble of nitrogen gas that develops in the vacuum created in the joint that is moved rapidly. The popping sound does not cause arthritis, just like cracking your knuckles does not cause arthritis. Chiropractic adjustments and movement should be painless. Physical therapists use manipulation to maximize motion of musculoskeletal structures, but they use more gradual motions to achieve the same outcome.

Scott, a thirty-four-year-old accountant, had surgery for a herniated disc. His leg pain improved but then recurred in six months and radiated down to the back of his thigh. Medication helped, but Scott wanted to decrease his need. He had six treatments with a chiropractor and had significant improvement in his back and thigh pain. This treatment allowed him to reduce his NSAID use to every other day—but he was not pain free.

Choosing a Chiropractor

Chiropractors may use manipulation alone or in combination with other complementary therapies. "Straight" chiropractors do only spinal manipulation; "mixers" use a variety of therapies—including nutritional supplements, homeopathic remedies, and acupuncture—to achieve balance in the nervous system. They often take X rays before beginning manipulation therapy. Many such X rays demonstrate slight curvatures, which may then be suggested as the cause of pain. However, the significance of these curvatures is questionable, because many people without back pain show similar degrees of curvature on spine X rays. Question the need for X rays before you begin treatment with a chiropractor, and see a medical doctor if you suspect any serious illness is causing your pain.

Make sure you choose a good chiropractor. While chiropractic treatment for low back pain is unlikely to harm you, injury is more likely if the practitioner has little understanding of the musculoskeletal system and the effects of adjustments on the lumbar spine.

You will know if a chiropractor is good if he or she:

- Takes time to listen to your problem
- Does not require X rays for treatment of acute low back pain
- Provides a timeframe for the course of therapy
- Treats only musculoskeletal disorders
- Lets you pay for one visit at a time
- Is willing to refer to a medical doctor if therapy is ineffective

Many chiropractors are affiliated with hospitals, health maintenance organizations, and large group practices, and you may also find a referral from friends and family. Just be sure to ask questions that provide information about the issues raised above.

Osteopathic Manipulation

Dr. Andrew Taylor Still developed the philosophy of osteopathic medicine because he believed in a unifying principle between body structure and function in health and disease. Still also believed physicians overlooked the body's ability to heal itself, a philosophy that was not accepted by allopathic (conventional) physicians in the late 1800s. Dr. Still started his own school of osteopathic medicine in 1892, and osteopathic schools soon were established throughout the United States. Today, the curriculum studied by osteopathic physicians (D.O.s) and allopathic physicians (M.D.s) is quite similar, but osteopaths also specialize in how disordered physical structures affect function. Allopathic and osteopathic physicians are licensed with similar rights and privileges.

The osteopathic physician observes abnormalities in structure, such as muscle spasm, restriction of motion, or sensitivity to palpation. The spine is considered the primary area of dysfunction because of its proximity to the autonomic nervous system, which monitors all the basic functions of the body. Osteopathic manipulation of the spine and other structures restores normal body mechanics and function, thereby restoring balance in the organ systems, including the nervous system. Improved function also results in improved blood flow. Osteopathic treatment may involve manipulation alone, a combination of manipulation and other complementary therapies, or drug therapy.

A variety of osteopathic techniques are available for the treatment of low back pain. Myofascial release, strain and counterstrain, cranial techniques (gentle manipulation of the head and spine), and manipulation with impulse (greater force) are some of the techniques that may be useful. Osteopathic manipulation has been shown to decrease back pain, but the benefit may be limited to a few weeks.

There are over fifty thousand osteopathic physicians in the United States, licensed through individual states; many belong to the American Osteopathic Association. Some D.O.s deliver only allopathic care; some D.O.s offer only certain forms of manipulation; and still others offer a wide variety of complementary therapies, too. Let your outlook for your back problem guide you in deciding if a D.O. offers therapy that will be helpful to you. And be sure to tell your osteopath if spinal manipulation increases your pain.

MASSAGE AND OTHER BODY WORK TECHNIQUES

The ancient Greek physician Hippocrates, the "father of medicine," believed that massage freed nutritive fluids to flow to the body's organs. The Romans further developed massage practices as part of their healing system. Eastern cultures in India and China have also developed massage techniques and promoted their benefits. Today we have various massage styles, mostly based on Eastern or Western techniques.

Western massage, such as Swedish massage, can relax tense muscles to improve range of motion, remove stress, and increase energy. The pressure on muscles brings a different sensation into the tissues and relieves pain. Chinese and Japanese forms of massage, such as shiatsu, improve the flow of energy (*qi*) through the body's energy channels (meridians). Pressure on acupuncture points releases blocked qi and restores the body's natural balance.

Reflexology

Reflexologists believe that the organs of the body have representations on different areas of the feet, hands, and ears. Thus, massaging reflex points on the feet and hands can influence vital organs in a distant location. The spinal column is located along the instep of the foot, for example. The spine is represented along the ear rim. By placing pressure on the reflex points, particularly in the feet, energy is released in the affected area, resulting in relaxation and pain relief.

Craniosacral Massage

This massage tries to balance the system that connects the skull (*cranio*) with the base of the spine (*sacrum*). Light touch is placed on the skull to balance muscle tension, and the sacrum may also be manipulated. This is gentle massage, with little risk of damaging underlying tissues.

Rolfing/Structural Integration

The theory behind rolfing, named for Ida Rolf, Ph.D., is that thickened fascia (the membrane covering your muscles) results from accumulated physical imbalances related to specific injuries, such as a hip strain. Connective tissue may shorten around the injury, which adds to unbalanced movements and postures. Rolfing is essentially a deep tissue massage technique involving vigorous movement to loosen adhesions of connective tissues covering these injuries. The technique can be painful as the tensions in joints, ligaments, and muscles are released. The therapy is given in ten one-hour weekly sessions.

How to Choose the Best Bodywork for You

Bodywork refers to a group of manual therapies that promote improved body mechanics and decreased stress. Get the most out of your bodywork technique by planning before your session in the following ways:

- Identify the goals of the technique you choose.
- Visit only an experienced practitioner.
- Tell the practitioner about your concerns.
- Rest after your session to enjoy its benefits.
- Talk with your therapist about any necessary preparation.

Massage techniques may use a light touch or a more vigorous stretching of muscles, so decide which type of massage you would most enjoy. Experienced bodywork therapists deliver the best sessions, so find a practitioner who knows the particulars of your condition and the useful techniques for your specific problem. Contact organizations that certify massage therapists or the licensing board of your state to determine the status of the practitioner you are considering. In addition, gather recommendations from other health professionals or the practitioner's patients.

ACUPUNCTURE

Acupuncture is based upon the Chinese theory that energy pathways, called meridians, carry the body's energy, which is known as *qi* or *chi*. Illness causes an imbalance in the flow of qi in the twelve primary meridians. Stimulation of specific points along the meridians can correct the flow of qi to optimize health or block pain. It also relieves pain through the release of endorphins. More than one million Americans use acupuncture on an ongoing basis, many of them because of musculoskeletal problems.

Traditional acupuncture uses thin needles at the 360 specific points along the meridians to rebalance the flow of energy. Between five and fifteen thin, flexible, solid, sterile needles are inserted from a mere fraction of an inch to four inches deep. As the needles are inserted, you may feel a range of sensations from a light needle prick to tingling, warmth, or pinching. The needles are left in place from five to sixty minutes (twenty minutes is about the average.) It may take a course of ten treatments to obtain maximum benefit, and you may need follow-up treatments, usually every few months, to maintain normal energy balance. In addition to needles, or in place of needles, practitioners may use heat, pressure, friction, suction, or electrical current connected to needles on acupuncture points. These may produce similar effects.

When a licensed practitioner does it, acupuncture has a good safety record. However, possible complications include infections (AIDS or hepatitis) if unsterile needles are used, organ punctures, dermatitis, and local bleeding. Make sure your therapist uses sterile disposable needles that are used only once so there is no chance of infection.

Acupuncture is an example of a complementary therapy that supplements the effectiveness of other treatments for chronic pain, including medications and physical therapy. As yet, we do not have good data on the frequency of a positive response to acupuncture treatments. It is worthwhile to try acupuncture if all other therapies have been tried but are not fully effective. Acupuncture should also be considered if toxic side effects prevent the use of medications.

A disadvantage is that the passive, time-consuming procedure is also relatively expensive since it is not yet universally covered by medical insurance, including Medicare.

YOGA AND OTHER BODY, MIND, AND SPIRIT TECHNIQUES

Currently popular in the West, yoga has its origin in Indian culture as part of the Ayurvedic form of therapy. The Sanskrit word "yoga" comes from the root *yug*, which means to join. Yoga is a philosophy of life that promotes awareness of the unity of the body, mind, and spirit. Patanjali, an Indian teacher, wrote about the principles of yoga thousands of years ago.

The postures (asanas) and breathing techniques (pranayama) closely associated with yoga in the Western world are means to increase physical strength and stamina needed for meditation. The harmony between physical and mental states brings greater self-awareness and health. In this context, yoga is both preventive and curative for ailments of the body, mind, and spirit.

In Western cultures, yoga postures have become the means to achieve better health, with a lesser emphasis on the mental aspect of meditation and self-realization. Yoga comes in many varieties. Most Westerners know the form called hatha yoga, combining *ha* for "sun," and *tha*, meaning "moon." Hatha yoga is the yoga of activity and is a disciplined system of gentle stretches and balancing exercises. Asanas, if done correctly, affect all the organs of the body. Postures are adjusted so that alignments are correct for the bones, joints, and organs. This proper alignment allows for the ideal function of the body.

The restorative powers of yoga to treat the kind of difficulties associated with back pain would seem an ideal fit. Many people who have learned the yoga postures report improvement in their pain and decreased stress.

The Stressed-Out Teacher

Alice, a forty-five-year-old elementary school teacher, had low back pain for two years. She could not remember what brought her pain on, but it was a real inconvenience because she had two children and a demanding job. Between her lesson plans and driving her children around to one event or another, she rarely took time to take care of her back, except when the pain became excruciating. Alice would take over-the-counter drugs until the pain lessened, and then she'd quit. She had no time for exercise, and she drank excessive amounts of caffeine during the day, which led to difficulty going to sleep at night.

This stressed-out teacher had many problems, one of which was her back. Eliminating the caffeine was only one of my suggestions, and she began taking an NSAID and started some simple stretching exercises. Her back improved, but she remained anxious and stressed. Alice told me that a friend of hers found yoga helpful for back problems and I encouraged her to go, not only to improve flexibility, but also to benefit from yoga's stress-relieving qualities.

After two years of participating in yoga exercise, Alice has less back discomfort and takes less medication. Equally important, she is much calmer, even though she still has responsibility for many children. Through yoga, Alice has learned to cope with her many stresses and she believes it has made a significant difference in the quality of her life.

Ideally, yoga should be done daily, and periodic classes allow for reinforcement of maintaining correct postures. Many exercise programs recommend rest days in between sessions, but yoga does not entail the kind of muscle strain and strenuous activity that makes rest necessary.

Under the guidance of an experienced teacher, you are at little risk of damage from exercises done correctly. Programs that build from the most safe and simple postures seem most appropriate. If a posture hurts, do not do it.

Choosing a teacher can be challenging. You don't need a license to teach yoga, and the philosophy of the teacher structures the class content and emphasis. Observe a class to determine if its objectives meet your needs. Then show illustrations of yoga postures to your physician and ask if any may be harmful to you.

Tai Chi

Tai chi is an ancient Chinese practice that gently moves the body through a number of slow, continuous, flowing postures. Unlike the martial arts, tai chi involves no impact or jarring motions. A session may last from twenty to sixty minutes and promotes deep breathing, balance, and stress reduction. There are five distinct styles of tai chi. Some do not require deep knee bending and would be ideal for those with back pain and knee arthritis.

Tai chi has been proven to be effective in improving musculoskeletal function. In a study of 215 people over age seventy, tai chi decreased their risk of falling compared to same age groups taught balance exercises and behavior modification. These people also had lower blood pressure and improved hand strength. Tai chi may help back pain by improving relaxation and regaining flexibility.

Tai chi is best learned from a teacher. It helps if the teacher has some appreciation of back pain and has had experience with students with this problem. Exercises should be done every day even for short periods of time. Exertion is not part of the process. Relaxation and stress reduction are part of the mental component of tai chi. Do not overlook it.

The Pilates Method

Joseph Pilates was a fitness trainer in Germany who emigrated to the United States in 1926. He developed "centrology," a system that incorporates the science and art of coordinated body-mind-spirit development through natural movements under strict control of the will. This method encompasses elements of Western and Eastern philosophy regarding the importance of motion and strength in the setting of inner calm and relaxation. Initially, Pilates was particularly popular with dancers like Martha Graham. More recently, with a growth in the number of Pilates studios and instructors, it has gained greater acceptance by the general public.

The program includes over five hundred different exercises designed to increase balance, flexibility, and strength by building more efficient muscles. Exercises are performed on a mat, a wall, or Pilates's apparatus including springs, barrels, and chairs. The program concentrates on strengthening abdominal, buttock, and spinal muscles. According to Sean Gallagher and Romana Kryzanowska, instructors of the Pilates Method, the six basic principles are concentration to movement, control of movement by the mind, strengthening the center of the body, flowing movement, precision, and proper breathing. Specific exercises are recommended for those with back pain.

A key to success with the Pilates Method is a well-trained and experienced teacher. Observation by an instructor can assure that your technique is correct. The number of teachers has grown but is limited to major cities in the United States and a few foreign countries. The website for instructors has updated information about instructors and their studios. Many of the exercises can be done on a mat without the use of an apparatus. Books and videos of the exercises are available for those who wish to try the conditioning program on their own.

MIND-BODY THERAPIES

Another form of complementary therapy is based upon the interaction between chronic pain and disease and psychological stress. Pain, when associated with a change in personality and thinking, may persist even after the original injury has healed. Negative emotions heighten pain and anxiety and increase muscle tension, and may lead to or exacerbate depression. Improving your emotional state has a beneficial effect on your physical status. Mind-body therapies include biofeedback, hypnosis, relaxation techniques, stress reduction, meditation, and guided imagery.

The therapies discussed below may increase your sense of self-control and accomplishment, but we do not all benefit from the same therapy. Investigate the techniques that appeal to you, and if one doesn't help, try another. These therapies have few side effects and are inexpensive, but they require time and effort. They may be used in combination with other therapies such as medications.

Biofeedback

Electronic monitors help you learn how to use your mind to control other body functions. Back pain often increases muscle tension, and surface EMGs can detect electrical signals generated by your muscles. The intensity of these signals is shown on a computer screen. The biofeedback practitioner teaches you how to use your mind to decrease the intensity of the muscle tension, which is shown on the computer as fewer signals. As you become more expert at the technique, you no longer need the EMG to confirm muscle relaxation, and you can do the technique any time without the equipment.

The key to success with biofeedback is persistence, because you need time to learn the technique. The advantages of biofeedback include lack of side effects and its portability—it travels wherever you go.

Hypnosis

Hypnosis is an altered state of awareness that allows you to narrow your attention and exclude extraneous stimulation. In the hypnotic state your intense concentration places your attention between wakefulness and deep sleep, to promote deep relaxation. In addition, pain may be decreased directly or may be transferred to another part of the body, or the type or quality of the pain may change to a sense of numbness or tingling. Initially, a hypnotherapist induces a hypnotic state, but you can learn techniques to hypnotize yourself and attain a trance.

Some psychiatrists utilize hypnosis as part of therapy, but other practitioners are not licensed. Before undergoing a session, inquire about the hypnotherapist's experience. Understand, too, that while you're suggestible in a hypnotic trance, you will not do anything that goes against your wishes. In other words, you remain in control.

Visualization

Visualization coaxes you to imagine your desired outcome. After relaxing with breathing exercises or progressive relaxation, focus your mind on specific sensations that are meaningful to you. To achieve a degree of pain relief, you might create an image of your muscle being its normal length or an image of the painful part or spot being swept away.

Jim, sixty-three, had left-sided low back pain and numbness in his foot while walking. He also had extensive practice in the martial arts and as a judo expert; he spent many hours focusing his thoughts on controlling his body as he performed judo. Jim's X rays indicated a narrowed neural foramen pressing on a nerve. Celebrex and stretching exercises improved his symptoms. One day, he told me about his visualization technique, which he believed helped relieve his pain. After completing breathing exercises, he focused his thoughts at the joint that had closed around his nerve. He visualized this joint opening up and relieving the pressure on his nerve. When his relaxation period was over, he realized that he could walk farther with less discomfort. His positive thoughts had helped bring about a good outcome, but he also understood that his visualization technique offered temporary relief, and he scheduled an MRI to determine the extent of his nerve compression.

Like relaxation techniques, visualization has no side effects and it is certainly cost-effective. Tapes are available to help you learn these techniques, and some provide guided visualization. In order to benefit from visualization you must decide if you believe that a mental function can have an effect on physical symptoms.

MEDITATION AND RELAXATION

Meditation is another technique that focuses the mind on a thought or sensation, and although we tend to associate meditation with Eastern philosophies and religion, the positive effects do not require religious or spiritual orientation. Focusing your mind on a single word or phrase can elicit the benefits of the relaxation response. Over time, silent repetition of a word or phrase can result in a change in consciousness. One of my patients explained the process by saying that meditation is not about falling asleep, but rather, is a silent concentration on thoughts, emotions, and sensations.

To meditate, you need a quiet place without distractions and a sitting posture that is comfortable and stable. (The crossed-legged lotus position is not necessary.) Meditation starts with deep breathing while focusing your thoughts on a meaningful word, phrase, or object. As every beginner knows, your mind will wander and "chatter," but the trick is sticking with the practice long enough to relax and improve concentration. Meditation reduces tension and helps relieve pain.

Relaxation Techniques

A variety of methods produce the relaxation response. Deep breathing exercises have the potential to calm the sympathetic nervous system, reduce blood pressure, and decrease pain. Many people do not know how to breathe deeply from the abdomen, but once learned, this type of breathing is a tool available at any time to help produce a relaxed state.

During relaxation exercises, deep breathing is done from the abdomen and chest in a reclining or flat body position. Place your hand over your abdomen as it rises while you inhale for a count of three; you will feel the abdomen "deflate" as you exhale over a count of three. You will notice changes in your body after only a few cycles, but I recommend starting with ten *slow* deep breaths. If you breathe too rapidly, you may become dizzy, so keep your breathing slow. Use this simple breathing exercise along with other relaxation techniques to decrease the intensity of pain.

Progressive muscle relaxation is a technique that contracts muscles and then relaxes them, starting with the feet and moving up through your legs, hips, buttocks, torso, arms, hands, chest, neck, and up to the muscles in the face. Many bookstores and natural food markets have a selection of audiotapes with instructions for a step-by-step "trip" through the body. Progressive relaxation exercises should be performed gently, with minimal contraction in muscles that are the source of discomfort.

Be aware of the amount of tension generated as you contract the muscles and remember that muscles that have not been exercised may cramp when you first begin practicing this technique. This type of exercise is a good way to acquaint yourself with your body—we tend to forget about all the muscles we need for normal movement. The last step is tensing and releasing all your muscles at once. Always end a session with deep cleansing breaths, which increase the level of relaxation.

Relaxation techniques are free of side effects; just be careful not to stand up too fast and become dizzy and risk a fall. These exercises involve minimal or no expense, but you must put in the effort to gain the benefit.

BODY SELF-AWARENESS

These techniques increase self-awareness of motions that increase pain and instability. Through improvement in movement, pain is decreased.

Alexander Technique

F. Mathias Alexander was an Australian actor whose voice was chronically hoarse whenever he went on stage. Ineffective medical therapies frustrated him, and he embarked on his own search for help. Alexander discovered that the misuse of the neuromuscular activity of his head, neck, and spine caused the vocal dysfunction. He corrected these problems by recognizing the tensions and inefficient use of his body, and eventually he taught his techniques to others.

In essence, the Alexander technique is a mind/body movement re-education course that heightens self-awareness of body movement and posture. The series of lessons demonstrates efficient ways to use painful joints and muscles so that movement takes less effort.

The Alexander technique is taught one-on-one in private lessons in which the teacher offers immediate feedback on harmful ways of holding and moving your body. A certified Alexander technique teacher is a highly trained professional who has completed sixteen hundred hours of training over a three-year period. Through the use of touch and words, the teacher coaches you to improve your standing, sitting, walking, bending, reaching, carrying, and lying down. Learning how to achieve balance with your own body goes along with an overall positive outlook. A course of therapy is about thirty private sessions, completed over fifteen weeks.

Feldenkrais Method

Moshe Feldenkrais, an engineer and martial arts expert, developed an awareness of movement as a method to overcome a knee injury. This method involves education about movements and stretches that make you more aware of your posture as you bend, sit, stand, or walk. The method retrains your muscles to avoid positions that cause pain. Group lessons go through a series of small movements to increase range of motion and flexibility. Individual sessions involve moving through ranges of motion that allow greater awareness of body flexibility. A set of lessons usually includes two sessions a week for six weeks.

MAGNET THERAPY

Many people, including some of my patients and some well-known sports figures, report remarkable relief of pain, sometimes with the first use of magnet therapy. Magnets are said to decrease muscle and joint pain, including back pain. They come in all shapes and sizes and are worn over the painful area. Magnets are placed in shoes, worn as necklaces, or are placed on beds like sheets.

However, we still don't understand how magnets are beneficial. We do know that static magnets do not make an electrical current unless they are passed though a coil of wire. Therefore, a stationary magnet on the skin would not be expected to generate a current. The mechanism that may play a role is the microcirculation in the blood vessels of the skin; this may generate the movement that results in an electrical current.

Numerous mechanisms have been suggested to explain why magnets work, including:

• Improved blood and lymph circulation
• Interference with superficial pain nerve fibers
• Stimulation of acupuncture points
• Increased production of endorphins, the body's natural pain relievers

To date, no scientific research has *proved* any of these mechanisms, and some studies show mixed results. Nevertheless, additional studies are underway.

The possible side effects associated with long-term magnet use have not been determined, but if magnets are effective by producing local electrical currents, they may be toxic if left in place for extended periods of time. For example, if magnets increase blood flow, they should not be used with acute injuries since increased blood flow will exacerbate swelling. If you have a pacemaker, don't use magnets, because they can cause irregular heartbeats.

Static magnets probably have the best chance of working on abnormalities and decreasing pain on the surface of the body, such as superficial muscle spasm. The deeper the abnormality, the less magnetic force will help. Currently, magnets appear to have little toxicity, so they are assumed to be safe. I recommend using only magnets that are marked with their strength and manufacturer. If your pain is not better after a few weeks or so, try another remedy.

Only one of my patients told me of positive results with magnet therapy. Melanie, age fifty-two, developed right leg sciatica secondary to a herniated disc, and since she did not respond to medical therapy, she underwent a discectomy. Her leg pain improved, but her low back pain and stiffness came back about four months after surgery and her thigh pain returned. Melanie improved with NSAID therapy and a muscle relaxant, and she had physical therapy for range of motion exercises. Within two months she had decreased pain and improved motion, and although initially she was reluctant to tell me why she was better, Melanie finally told me that she thought her magnets had done the trick. A friend had told her about magnets, and she had decided to get a corset with magnets in place. At first, there was no response, but within a few weeks her back was less painful and she was able to do her exercises. She could not be sure, but she thought her magnets had made the difference. I was not ready to disagree with her, and since there was no overt toxicity, I told her to continue with her magnets. Although her back pain has improved, she continues to wear her magnets.

My magnetic patient may have seen benefits from the therapy because the source of her pain was localized to superficial layers of the back. Deeper structures may not be reached by the magnetic forces generated by static magnets. These abnormalities (osteoarthritis of the lumbar spine) may be more resistant to magnet therapy.

HOMEOPATHY

Homeopathic remedies, developed at the end of the eighteenth century by Samuel Christian Hahnemann, a German doctor, are among the most frequently prescribed complementary therapies. One principle of homeopathy is "like cures like," meaning that a particular pattern of complaints can be cured by a drug that produces the same pattern of complaints in a healthy person. Another principle is that very small amounts of this drug have therapeutic value. The smaller the amount given, the greater the body's response. Some homeopathic drugs may be diluted to the degree that not even a single molecule of the original drug remains. In general, homeopathic remedies are believed to stimulate the body's ability to heal itself.

Homeopathic remedies may be tablets, liquids, or creams available from health food stores or pharmacies. These preparations contain so little medicine that most people can safely take them. You have little to lose when you try a homeopathic remedy if other therapies are not improving your back condition. But do tell your physician about these remedies. This advice is particularly important if your homeopathic practitioner recommends that you stop taking other medications. This could adversely affect your general medical condition, and remember that some medications should *not* be stopped abruptly.

NUTRITIONAL SUPPLEMENTS

An overwhelming number of nonprescription supplements line the shelves of health food stores and pharmacies. Many are made from plants and herbs that were remedies before pharmaceutical companies were able to create the modern array of drugs. Aspirin is an example of an enduring plant-based remedy made from willow tree bark, which was known to decrease fever, headache, and muscle pain. It served as a plant-based therapy long before its active chemical, salicin, was identified by German pharmacologists.

Manufactured drugs are produced under supervision of governmental agencies and are subjected to quality-control testing so you have assurance about their purity and dosage measurement. Dietary supplements are not regulated by the Food and Drug Administration, and an article from the *Washington Post* reported that a 1998 California investigation discovered that about one third of imported Asian herbals contained lead, arsenic, or mercury, or were spiked with drugs not listed on the label. In addition, without regulation, we don't know what part of the plant has the active ingredient, when it was harvested, or the storage conditions under which it was stored—all of which affect the potency. These issues have a direct effect on the usefulness of supplements you buy.

It's important to understand that not all "natural" plant therapies promote health—some plants are deadly. In books listing poisons, plants make up a significant number of agents that can stop the heart, cause low blood pressure, trigger convulsions, or result in coma. Never assume that "natural" is synonymous with "safe" or even "effective." Stick with plant remedies that have been subjected to research and testing.

Some dietary supplements offer complementary therapies to conventional interventions for acute and chronic low back pain. I always ask my patients to tell me if they are taking these supplements, because toxicities may occur in addition to or in spite of what the label on the bottle outlines. Don't start guessing about the possible cause of a new symptom when it could be related to a nutritional supplement.

Monitor your response in order to measure how you're doing. Has the pain decreased? Are you more functional? If the answers are yes, then increase your exercises and try to use less of your supplements over time. If the answers are no, then stop using the supplements and try something else.

The number of herbal supplements and their manufacturers continues to grow, which makes the choice of a single product difficult. Below are some guidelines that may be helpful:

- Choose a single supplement rather than a combination product; single agents have been studied, but the effects of combination products are more difficult to determine.
- Choose extracts over powdered preparations.
- Look for the FDA label describing the name and amount of supplement in the container.
- Choose products made by pharmaceutical manufacturers who are experienced in production of over-the-counter medications.

- Avoid products that describe miracle cures.
- Always take the supplement as described on the product label; if recommended doses are lacking or vague, don't take it.

Devil's Claw (Harpagophytum procumbens)

Harpagoside, the active ingredient of devil's claw, comes from the plant root. The plant is an appetite stimulant and mild analgesic; low back pain studies using this herbal remedy were conducted in Germany. In one study, 118 patients with low back pain were treated with 50 mg per day of harpagophytum extract. A greater number of patients receiving active extract were pain free when compared to the placebo group. In another study of 197 low back patients, a 100 mg dose of harpagophytum extract was found to be better than a 50 mg dose and placebo. Side effects included gastrointestinal symptoms, and the supplement is known to increase stomach acid secretion. Don't use it if you have a tendency to develop ulcers.

Ginger (Zingiber officinale)

Ginger is one of the herbs used in Ayurvedic medicine, the traditional medical system and philosophy of India. This spice has properties that inhibit PG production. By decreasing PGs, ginger has potential as an effective anti-inflammatory and analgesic substance. Studies of osteoarthritis and muscle pain have shown that ginger supplements are effective in decreasing pain. The therapy had no side effects and remained effective for up to thirty months. Ginger and other Ayurvedic herbs (turmeric, frankincense, ashwagandha) take a month or longer to have an effect. However, once established, the beneficial effect may last for an extended period measured in months to years, without increasing the dose.

If you take ginger or any of these herbs regularly, be sure to tell your doctor, because these herbs in large doses can interact with prescription medications. For example, ginger can increase the effect of blood pressure and blood thinning medications, thereby causing low blood pressure and bleeding.

Glucosamine and Chondroitin

These two supplements are promoted as treatments for osteoarthritis. Glucosamine sulfate, an aminosugar, which is a component of cartilage, has been available by prescription in Europe for years. Glucosamine comes from chitin, a substance extracted from the shells of crab, lobster, and shrimp. The usual allergy to shellfish is related to fish proteins, not the shells, so you should not be allergic to glucosamine even if you are sensitive to crab or shrimp. That said, a few of my patients have described sensitivity to glucosamine similar to what they experience with shellfish.

A Belgian study presented at the 1999 American College of Rheumatology meeting described glucosamine at a dose of 1500 mg per day as valuable in maintaining knee cartilage over a three-year period when compared to a placebo. However, problems with the X ray results have been raised, even though this study has been offered as positive data about the benefit of glucosamine for knee joints. No determination was made in this study about the effect of glucosamine on the lumbar spine. Cartilage in the knee is different from that in the lumbar spine end plates and discs, and glucosamine may not help disc disease. This point was made clear to me by one of my patients, with low back and knee pain.

Beth, seventy, had osteoarthritis of the knees and lumbar spine and had experienced symptoms for a number of years. I had treated her with Vioxx, which relieved pain symptoms in her knee and back. Prior to seeing me, Beth had been taking glucosamine sulfate for a number of months. Her knee pain improved but her back pain did not. Other patients have reported similar results.

I do not believe that glucosamine has a beneficial effect on back pain, but potential benefits for other joints currently are being studied. In addition, we do not have studies that report benefits or safety of glucosamine for more than a three-year time frame.

Chondroitin sulfate is a larger molecule than glucosamine and it may not be easily absorbed through the intestine and, thus, may not reach cartilage in joints. Cattle windpipes serve as the source of chondroitin used in supplements, because when derived from shark cartilage it may be contaminated with heavy metals such as mercury.

Chondroitin is taken 400 mg twice a day, but you may not see improvement for two months. Studies on chondroitin are fewer than those for glucosamine and any added benefit of chondroitin to glucosamine remains to be determined.

Chondroitin bears chemical similarity to heparin, a blood-thinning drug, so too many supplements may cause bleeding. If you bruise easily, or notice excessive bleeding when brushing your teeth, see your physician.

SAMe (S-adenosylmethionine)

Available in Europe since the 1970s, SAMe has been used to treat both arthritis and depression. It is a biochemical formed in the body from the essential amino acid methionine (found in proteins) and adenosine triphosphate, a major energy source in the body. The interaction of the two helps form cartilage.

Studies have reported improvement in depression and arthritis. It appears that SAMe decreases pain in osteoarthritis of the hands and may increase finger joint cartilage. In a study of thirty-six patients with osteoarthritis of the knee, hip, or spine, 1200 mg of SAMe per day or 1200 mg per day of ibuprofen, taken for four weeks, were equally effective in decreasing pain, and both had similar side effects.

We still do not have good data about the role of SAMe in the treatment of acute low back pain, or the long-term benefits and toxicities of SAMe. The downside of SAMe therapy is that it is a dietary supplement without FDA supervision. In addition, a breakdown product of SAMe is homocysteine, associated with cardiac health risks.

MSM: Methylsulfonylmethane

MSM is a derivative of dimethyl sulfoxide (DMSO), the chemical used to protect human tissues when they are frozen. It is also used in its medical-grade form to treat a bladder condition, interstitial cystitis. DMSO is a solvent passing molecules across membranes such as the skin and has been reported to cause fogging of the lens in the eyes of laboratory animals given the compound over extended periods of time. It also leaves a bad taste in the mouth and gives off a garlic aroma.

MSM has none of the bad characteristics of DMSO, including the garlic aroma. MSM does not require a prescription like DMSO does, since MSM is a dietary supplement. To date, no specific studies for MSM in low back pain have been conducted. MSM may take up to a month to work, and it appears that MSM isn't particularly helpful for acute low back pain. On the other hand, MSM may be beneficial as a complementary therapy for people with chronic low back pain. MSM comes as a 500 mg capsule. The recommended maximum dose per day should be found on the pill container. The side effects associated with a higher dose include diarrhea and cramps. If no effect is seen by the end of the second month on MSM, stop using it.

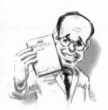

DR. B'S PRESCRIPTION SUMMARY

R

- Complementary therapy should not replace conventional therapy.

- Tell your doctor about any complementary therapies, because they may conflict with or have an adverse effect on conventional treatment.

- Manual therapies such as chiropractic manipulation or massage can sometimes help decrease muscle pain.

- Mind-body therapies can help decrease stress through relaxation

- Acupuncture is now more widely accepted by conventional medecine as a way to offer additional pain relief.

Dr. B—

10

WHAT TO KNOW BEFORE YOU CONSIDER SURGERY

Spine surgery always is a trauma to your back. Even minimally invasive surgeries damage your skin, muscles, blood vessels, and discs, so healing takes time. In addition, surgery means that you no longer have all the pieces of your spine that you were born with, a situation that puts added pressure on the parts that remain. Alterations in spinal anatomy from surgery may be minimal or they may significantly modify the function of your spine. And the results of surgical intervention do not end when you are wheeled into the recovery room. For the rest of your life, the effects of surgery can unfold.

The United States has the highest number of spinal surgeries per capita in the world. European countries such as Sweden have fewer. Swedish surgeons are paid a salary independent of the number of the surgeries they perform, whereas in the United States many spinal surgeons are paid for each operation. This payment system encourages surgeons to consider operative solutions at an earlier point in the course of recovery. Some regions of the United States have higher rates of back surgery than others. The existing bias toward surgery may be related to experience of local surgical training programs toward earlier surgical intervention. However, a decrease in insurance preauthorization approvals and lowered reimbursement levels is reversing this trend.

UNDERSTANDING THE RISKS

Every year hundreds of thousands of men and women undergo lumbar spine surgery because of low back and leg pain. The vast majority of these surgeries are appropriate and for most people the surgical outcome is excellent, but unfortunately we cannot say that surgery is successful 100 percent of the time.

A small but significant percentage of spine surgery patients have outcomes that are less than ideal, including:

- Wrong operation for the spinal disorder
- Wrong surgical site
- Inadequate surgical correction
- Inexperienced surgeon
- Postoperative complications
- Anesthetic death

Most people do not think about these things when they choose surgery, although they do have some degree of fear. Surgeons are obligated to get your "informed consent" before they operate, and so they must describe the benefits and risks of each procedure. However, most people are focused on relieving their pain, and the human tendency is to think that bad outcomes happen to other people. Think again.

When Surgery Is the Wrong Choice

The days of exploratory back surgery are over. Now that we have new radiographic techniques, almost all back anatomy can be visualized without invading the body. A decision to undergo surgery should never arise from a sense of desperation. Consider all the facts first. For example, if your disc herniation is on the opposite side of your leg pain, then it is not the cause of your sciatica. Removing that disc will not help your pain. Remember our guideline: Lumbar disc surgery is for leg pain, not back pain.

Surgery is questionable when pain or weakness has been present for months or years. A loss of function for years is not an indication for surgery because an operation does not lead to improved function. A surgical research project took a group of patients with stable neurologic deficits and operated on half of them. After three years, the nerve damage was similar in both the non-surgical and surgical groups. In a stable situation, surgery is performed to achieve pain relief, not to improve function.

Do not have an operation just because you were injured at work and other employees have had a similar procedure. What worked for others may not apply to your situation, and an operation can seriously delay your return to work. In addition, be certain that the procedure is in your best interests and not those of your employer or physician.

Is Surgery Right for You?

Surgery is indicated only if the clinical findings of leg pain correlate with physical findings and radiographic abnormalities. The specific cause of sciatica must be identified, and possible systemic disorders must be eliminated as potential causes of your back pain. In addition, MRI or CT findings must identify the correct anatomic level of disc herniation. Finally, you must understand the procedure and believe the benefits outweigh the risks. If all these factors coincide, surgery has an excellent chance of being successful.

Once you make the decision to undergo surgery, you must choose the best procedure to achieve the best results with the least risk for a bad result or complications.

These days, a number of new technologies such as laparoscopes and lasers are used for spinal procedures. While these technologies are amazing, they are new, and accumulated experience is naturally more limited when compared to the more tried-and-true spinal surgical techniques. If you consider a new technique, be sure your surgeon has had extensive training and experience using it. In addition, you should know if the procedure is experimental or is actually an old technology being used in a new way. Of course, find out why the new technique is better than older, time-tested procedures for your particular situation.

The Biblical Scholar

Father Mark, a fifty-six-year-old priest and biblical scholar, was having difficulty completing a book he was writing. At first he had difficulty with using his arms while sitting at his computer, and even lifting them to waist level caused severe pain. Naturally he was concerned that he would no longer be able to type. His first diagnosis was bilateral tennis elbows, and elbow bands and arm strengthening exercises allowed him to return to his computer to finish the first volume of his book.

The problem with his back started when he began the second volume, which put him in front of his computer for longer periods. Eventually he noticed increasing back and leg pain, which, at the beginning, was only in one side of his back. Standing up improved his pain, but his work demanded more time at the computer, which increased pain and progressively involved his buttock, his calf, and his foot. Eventually he was writing less and standing more. NSAIDs helped decrease pain, but his gastrointestinal tract did not tolerate these medications. An MRI scan revealed a herniated disc compressing the sciatic nerve, resulting in back and leg pain. Epidural corticosteroid injections were helpful but not curative, so after great soul searching, Mark decided to undergo a discectomy (partial removal of the herniated disc) and a foraminotomy (enlargement of the exit for the spinal nerve). The operation was a success, and he had almost immediate relief of his leg pain. Postsurgical back pain lasted about four weeks, and after six weeks he was back at his computer.

Our biblical scholar had a good result from his surgery and has continued to be pain free, so for him, surgery was the right decision.

Making the Descision

Keeping this background information in mind, you can begin to measure the risks and benefits of spinal surgery and determine if you are among the estimated 2 to 5 percent of people with back and leg pain who need surgery. In some circumstances, surgery can help those with sciatica feel better faster than medicines alone. For example, patients with nonoperative therapy for herniated discs have the same long-term outcomes (over a period of ten years) as those who have surgery, but the surgical group has more rapid relief of symptoms.

You may be a candidate for spinal surgery if you have:

- Bowel or bladder incontinence (CEC syndrome)
- Progressive muscle weakness with a foot drop, or you are unable to walk on your heels or raise your toes—your weakness may reverse spontaneously, but the longer the weakness remains, the less likely it is that strength will return
- Resistant, severe sciatica
- Recurrent, incapacitating sciatica—you may have one sciatica attack that completely resolves, but soon after, pain down the leg returns and becomes increasingly severe; if the frequency and intensity of attacks interfere with your ability to work or enjoy typical activities of daily living, surgery is a worthwhile choice. In general, surgery is indicated when you experience a third recurrence of sciatica.

DISCECTOMY

Open discectomy is the gold standard of spinal surgery and can initially bring good to excellent results in up to 95 percent of patients, provided they are appropriate candidates for the procedure. Minor complications occur in 4.7 percent of cases and the mortality rate is 0.03 percent.

This technique requires a three-inch incision in your back to expose the area of disc herniation and nerve compression and requires spinal or general anesthesia. Only the portion of the disc that is protruding and compressing the nerve is removed. The remainder of the disc is left in place to continue its work as a shock absorber. Extra bone may be excised (laminectomy) if the nerve is constricted in the spinal canal.

Microdiscectomy

Microdiscectomy involves a one-inch incision, a high-magnification surgical microscope, and intense illumination. The advantages are improved visualization of the anatomy, less bleeding, and less trauma to the muscles in the spine. The success rate for microdiscectomy to relieve leg pain is 90 percent. The technique offers more rapid recovery time, earlier discharge from the hospital, and generally an earlier return to work.

However, this technique is not without concerns. Recurrence of disc herniation and tearing of the covering of the spinal canal (dura) occur more frequently with microdiscectomy. If the dura tears, the spinal fluid leaks out. This can cause headaches. Additionally, with a smaller incision, it is more likely the surgeon will not see pieces of disc or some nerve compression that has moved from the original location of the herniation. For this reason, a second operation often becomes necessary. Make sure your surgeon has extensive experience with microdiscectomy and firmly believes it will help you.

Percutaneous Discectomy

Percutaneous discectomy is called the Band-aid Surgery. It is based on the premise that decompression of the nerve root can be achieved indirectly by entering the central portion of the disc and decreasing its volume, thereby resulting in the retraction of the disc herniation. Alternatively, if disc herniation is in an exposed position, not covered by vertebral bone, a probe placed through the skin during an X ray visualization can remove it. A tiny (one-centimeter) incision allows the entry of a surgical probe, and sedation and local anesthesia is all you need during the procedure. Once the procedure is completed, a Band-aid covers the wound, thus the name.

Percutaneous suction discectomy removes the central disc material with a rotary blade and the pieces of the disc are vacuumed up through the probe. Some have reported a success rate as high as 85 percent, but others remain skeptical. Percutaneous procedures have been challenged by findings based on MRI studies that revealed no significant change in the appearance of the postsurgical herniated disc in the area of protrusion.

Percutaneous laser discectomy uses a laser at the end of the probe to vaporize the central portion of the disc. Laser energy is converted to heat in the disc tissues, which results in decreased volume of the gel in the disc. The procedure, which requires only local anesthesia, has reported improvement in about 75 percent of patients. The primary concern is achieving the appropriate amount of laser energy. Too much laser energy can damage surrounding tissues such as the nerve, vertebral endplates, or facet joints. This damage may then be a cause for chronic low back pain from a different source.

SPINAL FUSION

It would be wonderful if we needed only Superglue to get the bones to stick together. Unfortunately, a lumbar fusion is more complicated. The surface of the bone that is going to be fused is roughened so that a repair response is started. Then the surgeon places a new piece of your own bone, which is taken from your pelvic bone, to fuse over the roughened bone. Alternatively, allograft is used. This is bone taken from those who have left their bodies for medical science. Bone banks carefully screen bone donors for infectious illnesses, including AIDS and hepatitis. Using allograft means that a second incision in your body is not needed in order to have enough bone for a fusion. Sometimes the donor site for the fusion is more painful than the lumbar surgical site.

The basic idea behind a fusion is that your own bone cells will replace the graft bone over a six-to-twelve month period, during which time you will be in a spinal brace while the fusion "takes." The living fusion will become solid, offering stability to that segment of the spine. Sometimes the fusion may be augmented with metal hardware (see below) for added stability.

Fusion surgery is complicated and it doesn't always work. The nonunion—where the fusion didn't take—may be a source of pain, independent of the original cause for the operation.

Current orthopedic research is looking at new ways to fuse bones. Certain bone proteins, when sprinkled on areas prepared for fusion, are able to get significant production of bone without the need for donor-site bone. When these are available, the success rate for fusion will increase.

Studies have demonstrated that one's overall health—not age—is the essential factor in deciding who is a candidate for spinal stenosis surgery. So, if you're in good general health, your age should not be an impediment to enjoying a better quality of life through surgery.

SPINAL INSTRUMENTATION: THE HARDWARE STORE

The exhibit area at today's spinal surgery meetings looks like your neighborhood hardware store—one can wander around and examine a vast array of drills, hammers, screws, plates, and rods. This hardware can be placed in the spine with the intention of decreasing pain, improving function, and limiting instability. Spinal instrumentation is particularly important in people who have sustained significant trauma to the spine. Spinal rods can immediately stabilize fractures of the spine, and hardware can straighten scoliotic curves. On occasion, the bone grafted for fusion is stabilized with the addition of rods to decrease movement. Pedicle screws and cages, which are spacers between discs, are among the new hardware used to improve spinal conditions. Currently, experimental testing is under way on an artificial disc.

If you are considering surgery now, you need to know that your surgeon is familiar with the instrumentation used in your operation and that the hardware has been specifically designed for this problem and has a track record for reliability. Before the instrumentation is initially placed, you and your surgeon need to discuss the potential need to remove the hardware. You might assume that hardware in the body must cause pain, but that isn't the case. Once healing has occurred, the hardware causes no pain and you can function normally. Medical scientists are always developing new techniques and instrumentation to improve spinal care. Be sure you know the purpose of the procedure and the hardware, because it is always easier to leave hardware out than retrieve it later.

The Five-Level Man

Juan, sixty, asked my advice about the deterioration of his back. His RA had been well controlled for over a decade, and the disease had not limited his activities. In fact, Juan still ran regularly, played tennis three times a week, and went hiking on vacations. However, while his RA was fine, his back was not, and he had developed increasing left thigh pain and numbness. NSAIDs, narcotic analgesics, and epidural injections had diminished his pain but had not completely relieved it. Naturally he was frustrated because he was unable to do any of his recreational exercise.

X ray evaluation revealed multiple levels of severe disc degeneration from L-1 to L-2 and L-4 to L-5. An orthopedic surgeon evaluated Juan about his back pain and severe limited motion. After extensive discussions, a five-level laminectomy with fusion with five-level rod placement was completed. A postoperative infection was treated with antibiotics. After ten months he was walking four miles every day and was ready to start running on a treadmill. Juan does not regret his decision to undergo surgery. As an aside, his RA has remained under control and his arthritis regimen has not hindered recovery from his fusion operation.

EMERGENCY SURGERY

Cauda equina compression syndrome (CEC) is a rare problem, but one that needs immediate spinal surgery. CEC causes bladder and bowel incontinence, loss of sensation between the legs (saddle anesthesia), and bilateral sciatica. This occurs when a large herniated disc compresses nerve roots at the end of the spinal canal, the cauda equina. CEC may also be caused by an infection in the epidural area or bleeding from blood-thinning medication. Pressure on the nerves causes the loss of neurologic functions, such as the ability to control the bladder and bowels. Control will not return unless pressure is taken off the nerve. Therefore, it's essential to remove the compression as quickly as possible.

CEC patients should receive immediate MRI evaluation of the spine to identify the cause and location of compression. They have little choice but to go forward with surgery to return neurologic function. The best results occur if surgery is performed within forty-eight hours. However, the decompression surgery should take place even if the compression has been present for days. Studies have demonstrated the slow return of neurological function with decompression surgery despite extended periods of CEC.

ANTERIOR SPINE SURGERY

Most lumbar spine surgery is approached from the surface of the back, through the muscles, to the posterior portion of the vertebra. Operations that relieve compression of the nerves by the discs or joints can be carried out by this posterior approach. On occasion, an anterior approach through the abdomen to reach the front of the spine is necessary. Fusion of the lumbar spine can be accomplished in this manner. An anterior approach allows for the placement of bone between the vertebrae to form an interbody fusion. This approach may allow a greater opportunity for a successful result and improved mechanics of the spine but is associated with a greater number of possible complications. The intestines may be irritated by the procedure and may not work normally for days. Blood clots may occur more often in association with this approach. You should choose a surgeon with experience with this technique if you require this form of fusion operation.

CHOOSING AN ORTHOPEDIC SURGEON OR NEUROSURGEON

I've had the good fortune to work with excellent spine surgeons, and both orthopedists and neurosurgeons gain experience with these operations. Orthopedists with an interest in spine surgery usually take extra training to gain greater expertise with spinal procedures. Neurosurgeons may not learn about spinal instrumentation or fusion, but they have expertise in procedures that preserve spinal cord function. Either type of experienced spinal surgeon can perform the typical discectomy, laminectomy, or decompression operation. If a fusion or instrumentation is required, an orthopedic surgeon should be part of the surgical team.

If you want the best chance for a good surgical outcome, then choose your spine surgeon carefully. This sounds logical, but the process may not be so obvious. As you know, surgery is subspecialized into different parts of the body. In order to gain experience, spine surgeons have extra years of training in the techniques used to fix fractures, straighten curves, remove pieces, and fuse them together. Here are some characteristics of good spine surgeons. They are:

• Board-certified in a surgical specialty
• Recommended by your primary care physician or internist
• Recommended by a person you trust who had spine surgery
• Able to communicate with you about your surgery
• Extensively experienced with the procedure you require

Ask questions. You need confidence in your surgeon, and you should understand your procedure:

• How (and why) will it improve my condition?
• How long will it take to heal from my surgery?
• What are the potential surgical complications?
• Do my other medical conditions affect the success of the procedure?

You may not like the answers to these questions, but your surgeon should answer them before you have the surgery. If the surgeon doesn't want to speak with you before the procedure, it won't be any easier after the surgery. Always consider a second opinion, even if you are satisfied with your initial surgeon.

If your car needs bodywork you get two estimates before you would proceed. Surely your body is worth two "estimates." If both physicians agree on the need for surgery and the operative procedure, you can feel reassured. If they don't agree, at least you will be educated about differences of opinion. If you go to a neurosurgeon for the first opinion, try an orthopedic surgeon for the second. You can then decide which procedure makes the most sense to you.

Preoperative Evaluation

Once you decide to have surgery, an evaluation is completed to determine your health status before the operation. You will have blood tests, including a test for clotting factors; an electrocardiogram; and depending on your age or smoking history, a chest X ray may be required. The older you are, the more tests you undergo. These evaluations identify potential problems that may occur during or after your operation.

Conditions such as diabetes, angina, high blood pressure, and so forth influence the way the anesthesiologist willl treat you during surgery, and they affect your post-operative treatment as well. For example, you will stop taking baby aspirin to help prevent cardiovascular disease, and if you take an NSAID, you will stop one to four weeks before the surgery, depending on how long the drug stays in your body.

If you are taking one of the new COX-2 inhibitors, you may not need to discontinue your medicine until the time of surgery. This is possible because the COX-2 inhibitors rofecoxib and celecoxib do not interfere with the ability of platelets to stop bleeding.

Depending on the extent of the surgery, you may want to donate one or two units of blood; if a multilevel procedure is planned, two units is appropriate. Banking your blood decreases the risk of being exposed to infectious illnesses, even though they are rarely transmitted through blood transfusions.

If you smoke and have wanted to quit, now is a good time. Decreased lung function decreases oxygen to the tissues that are trying to heal. If you are having a fusion operation, smoking will increase the risk of nonunion. Smoking also increases the risk for lung infections. Some surgeons will insist on your quitting smoking before scheduling an elective fusion procedure.

Plan for your needs when you return home after surgery. If you live alone, prepare an area that will be comfortable and that has a clear path with no rugs on the floor between your chair and the bathroom. And speaking of the bathroom, renting a raised toilet seat can do wonders for making one of life's necessities a bit easier. In addition, try to prepare meals ahead of time and have them on hand in your freezer so you don't have to think about cooking.

YOUR HOSPITAL STAY

Once you have had approval from your insurance carrier and the date has been set, you will enter the hospital. Unless you have multiple medical problems, you'll be seen the day of your operation. You will sign an informed consent form stating that you understand the benefits and risks of the procedure, but do not sign this form unless you are satisfied with the information you have received from your physician.

The anesthesiologist will evaluate your medical history and allergies, if they are an issue. The anesthesiologist and surgeon will decide on spinal versus general anesthesia. During the procedure, you will receive an intravenous catheter to receive fluids and medications. If general anesthesia is used, medicine is given by vein to relax you while a tube is placed in your windpipe to control your breathing. If spinal anesthesia is used, a needle is placed in the spinal canal through which medication is delivered, and you will remain awake for the procedure.

After the surgery, you will be observed in the recovery room to be sure you are stable. Pain medicines for the postoperative period are initiated, first through a patient controlled analgesia (PCA) pump. The amount of medicine is controlled, but you can deliver it through the vein as you need it. Studies have demonstrated that when you have control over the timing of the pain medication, less is used than the amount you would receive when the medication is scheduled, and you obtain greater comfort.

You will be sent home from the hospital when you can eat and get out of bed. You will probably be stiff and have difficulty walking, but this is expected, particularly if you have had an open procedure.

AFTER SURGERY—THE HARD PART

The most difficult part of the surgical process occurs after the operation when you reenter normal life. In the perioperative period, care must be taken with the surgical wound so that it heals without developing an infection. A nurse will generally discuss wound care before you are discharged from the hospital. Analgesic medications, some of which are narcotic, are generally useful as you get used to doing daily activities for yourself.

To regain maximum function, you must move around. Initially, your body will try to keep all the cut tissues as still as possible to allow for healing. However, you must move these tissues to improve blood flow, which facilitates healing. At the beginning, movements are slow and small and repeated only a few at a time. As pain and time allow, you'll increase your movements.

Your goal is to obtain maximum motion with minimal pain.

Physical Therapy

Physical therapy is part of your postoperative treatment. Physical therapists may seem to be mean taskmasters, but their expertise encourages you to improve your functioning in a sheltered environment. These health care professionals are trained to help you with normal activities, and they guide you in how long to sit or stand. Physical therapists can also help with comfortable positions to sleep at night. You also will learn how to get in and out of a car in the easiest way. In addition, physical therapists teach ways to perform various chores while limiting stress on the back. However, you should ask your doctor about performing more strenuous tasks such as mowing the lawn or vacuuming the carpets.

Give Yourself Time to Heal

Although we would like to think in terms of weeks, healing within months is a more realistic goal. Getting better is hard work, and what once was done with very little energy seems like a major task now. I often tell patients to count to ten when they become frustrated by their limitations. This pause allows them to think about the way their back pain used to be. At least now they are on the road to recovery. In all likelihood, your recovery will take the same course as that taken by the vast majority of people who undergo successful back surgery.

FAILED BACK SURGERY SYNDROME

Although spine physicians do not like to admit failure, they must acknowledge the group of patients who do not improve with their first back surgery. (Within all surgical groups, some patients do not improve.) If the pain was never improved, the initial surgery may have been done at the wrong level or the procedure may have been inadequate to reverse the abnormal anatomic changes. A second possibility is that another disc herniation has occurred at the same level. The latter group usually have a pain-free period before their leg pain returns. People with one herniated disc are at greater risk for another, and they may have a new disc herniation at a different spinal level. Those with pain primarily in the back may have instability because the laminectomy may have been too extensive. Others develop a scar around the operative site surrounding the decompressed nerve. Back and leg pain may occur six to twenty-four months after the initial operation.

Another operation may help correct these abnormalities. However, another surgical procedure will not alter the progression of arthritis or change the development of scar tissue. For this, you need nonsurgical management. Scar tissue (epidural fibrosis) removal through direct visualization remains experimental. In addition, the primary difficulty is not the removal of the scar but rather the means to control the inflammatory process so that no additional scar returns in the location where the original scar was removed. Epidural fibrosis remains a perplexing chronic disorder.

When you consider a second or third spinal operation, consult with a spinal surgeon who has experience with patients who have had multiple spinal surgeries. Physicians with this experience can make the difficult decisions about the potential benefits of another spine operation versus a nonoperative course. Everyone's usual tendency is to want to do *something* to make the situation better, and it takes mature experience to say no when others want to do a procedure even though it is more likely to harm than to help.

FUTURE SURGICAL TREATMENTS

Currently, researchers are investigating three new procedures for the treatment of disc degeneration and vertebral body collapse. These invasive techniques have been helpful to people with back pain, but their long-term safety remains unproven.

Intradiscal electrothermal annuloplasty (IDET) is used for painful discs. An electrothermal catheter is threaded inside the disc. Released energy "cooks" the collagen in the disc like an egg, and the disc becomes stiff and loses its cushioning properties. However, patients are reported to have less back pain after this procedure. The exact mechanism that brings about the improvement is not yet clear. Only a small number of individuals have had this procedure, with only short-term follow-up. We need longer follow-up periods before we can confidently recommend this procedure.

Vertebroplasty and kyphoplasty are two new procedures for acute compression fractures of the spine that cause severe low back pain which may be resistant to bracing and narcotic analgesic. Using a fluoroscope for visual guidance, the surgeon can inject bone cement into the vertebra. The cement supports the fractured vertebra and relieves pain. There are potential complications. For example, using too much pressure will fracture the thin wall of the vertebral body. In addition, radicular leg pain also may be a complication, and it may be necessary to surgically remove the injected bone cement.

With kyphoplasty a tube with a balloon at the end is threaded through a needle into the vertebral body. The balloon is inflated and the vertebral body's shape is reestablished. The balloon is removed and the space is filled with cement pushed in with low pressure. With this procedure there is much less risk for the cement to escape through the bone into the spinal canal. Kyphoplasty relieves pain associated with osteoporotic fractures in a short period of time. This procedure is successful when undertaken within six weeks of the vertebral body fracture. While this procedure is experimental, it is undergoing clinical trials, and long-term follow-up is needed in order to identify potential complications of this intervention over time.

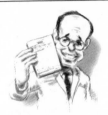

DR. B'S PRESCRIPTION SUMMARY

R

- 5 percent of back patients require spine surgery.

- Over 90 percent of spine surgeries are successful.

- The first surgery for a herniated disc or spinal stenosis has the best chance of success.

- Remember, disc surgery is for leg pain, not back pain.

- When a back injury or degenerative condition causes loss of bowel or bladder function, leg weakness, or intolerable pain, immediate surgery is usually necessary.

- Before you agree to surgery, always ask questions about the short- and long-term side effects, and be sure your surgeon has extensive experience treating others like you.

Dr. B—

PART THREE:
LIVING WITHOUT BACK PAIN

11

LOWER YOUR RISK FOR BACK PAIN WITH PREVENTION

The concept of prevention does not have a great track record, and this dismal situation is true not only for back pain but for most health issues. It's really quite simple. Healthy people lack motivation to participate in preventive activities. They wait until they have their back attack (or other illness) and then try to prevent a recurrence.

Once you have had one back attack, you are at greater risk of having another within a year. Some studies suggest this is true for as many as 50 percent of back pain sufferers. However, the second attack is usually milder than the first. The second attack occurs because people forget the lessons learned from the first back pain episode. They go back to their old habits and lift objects from awkward positions, stretch too far, or sit too long.

Do not become a repeat back offender. Remember what caused your first back attack. Practice good body mechanics, rest when appropriate, and exercise at the correct time of the day (generally later in the day). If you follow these simple rules, a second attack of pain is less likely. Here are my guidelines for avoiding back problems—and preventing them from recurring.

LIFESTYLE CHANGES

Don't Smoke

If you are a smoker, make every effort to stop now—your back, along with your lungs and heart and other organs, too, will thank you. All the tissues of the body require oxygen to maintain their function, and smoking robs these tissues—especially your spinal discs—of the optimal amount of oxygen. Because no blood vessels supply the interior of the discs, all the oxygen has to seep in from the surface. If the blood contains less oxygen, the discs receive less, too, and lack of oxygen is part of the disc disintegration process that increases the risk of herniation.

Maintain Fitness

When you are physically fit you are at less risk for developing low back pain. We can define fitness in a number of ways. For example, cardiovascular fitness is the ability to climb stairs or run without getting short of breath. In a study of fire fighters, those in good physical condition had significantly decreased risk of back pain compared to those in poor physical condition.

Strong back muscles represent another type of fitness. Compared to other muscles in the body, the muscles in the back are generally weak; if we increase strength in these muscles, we can decrease our risk of developing low back pain. While this is important for everyone, it is essential for those whose jobs require heavy lifting and physical labor. Exercises that strengthen the muscles in the front (abdominal flexors) and in the back (back extensors) can decrease your risk of injury if you lift heavy objects or twist and bend frequently while at work.

Do your general fitness exercises every other day. The day off allows your body to revitalize muscles fatigued by the exercise. Engage in an exercise program vigorous enough to stimulate about thirty minutes of perspiration. "Breaking a sweat" means you have used enough calories to generate heat, which is a sympathetic nervous system response that benefits the part of the nervous system that inhibits pain. These types of exercise also improve circulation, flexibility, and muscle tone.

Maintain a Good Body Weight

Obesity in itself is not a risk factor for the development of low back pain, but it prevents you from doing exercises properly and comfortably. If obesity results in a sedentary lifestyle, then all the risks associated with inactivity remain present. For most people, the body mass index (BMI) is a good measure for whether or not you are overweight. For example, if you are six feet tall and weigh 200 pounds, your BMI would be 27, which is a bit high. You would do better at a weight of 170 or 180. If you are five-foot-five and weigh 150 pounds, you would have a BMI of 25. Guidelines from the National Institutes of Health define overweight as a BMI greater than 25. Obesity starts at a BMI of 30.

Get Plenty of Antioxidants in Your Diet

Make sure your diet contains abundant amounts of fruits and vegetables, which are good sources of vitamins A, C, and E, the antioxidants. Beta-carotene is found in green and yellow fruits and vegetables like cantaloupe, apricots, spinach, and carrots. Dairy products and eggs provide vitamin A, citrus fruits are loaded with vitamin C, vegetable oils supply vitamin E.

Scientific evidence proving the direct benefit of antioxidants on intervertebral discs is still lacking. Although I do not have the clinical trials to prove it, I believe that antioxidant supplements have the potential to slow oxidative damage to the spine. Discs of the spine are one of the places that might benefit from this therapy. An adequate dose of antioxidants, preferably from food, is important to maintain spine health.

Our exposure to free radicals is part of the ongoing aging process throughout the body, including the spinal discs. In an autopsy study of people aged thirteen to eighty-six, oxidative damage was identified in cartilage cells in the middle of the discs. The damage started in the teenage years and continued in each age group. In addition, evidence of the body's attempts to repair the oxidative damage was present in all examined discs. This study confirmed the notion that disc degeneration from oxidative damage starts in the second decade of life.

These active oxygen molecules (free radicals) attach to cells in your spinal discs and cause damage. The cells try to repair the injuries but are ineffective, which means the disc wears out too soon. Antioxidants (vitamins E, A, C, and beta-carotene) are able to neutralize the damaging effects of oxygen radicals.

If you take these nutrients as supplements, keep in mind that the fat-soluble vitamins A and E are absorbed and stored with fat and thus are eliminated very slowly. Excessive amounts can accumulate in the body and become toxic. Health problems associated with taking these antioxidant supplements at levels above the recommended limits include kidney stones and diarrhea with vitamin C, increased bleeding in people taking anticoagulant medicines with vitamin E, and hair and nail breakage with selenium. Doses of vitamin A at a level of 100,000 units are toxic. The National Academy of Sciences has recently set "upper intake levels" for vitamins C and E and the mineral selenium as follows:

- Vitamin C: 2,000 mg
- Vitamin E: 1,100 mg (synthetic)
- Selenium: 400 mcg

USE GOOD BODY MECHANICS

The spine is a beautifully engineered structure, and we know posture is good if someone can effortlessly maintain normal position and movement for extended periods of time. Maintaining normal posture is a function of the ligaments that support the spine and legs and also of normal tension in muscles. When any component of the balanced spine is moved off center, this effortless state is altered (fig 11.1).

Every day, your spine enables you to accomplish a number of tasks without pain. Think of it. Your spine supports your body when you lift a large object, and it stays straight when you make it sit in a car on a drive from Washington, D.C., to Boston, with only one stop for gasoline. If your spine is positioned correctly while you accomplish these tasks, you will suffer no ill effects. However, if a heavy load is off center, which twists your back, or if the car seat offers no support, you will probably develop back pain.

If I had to choose the one position that causes the most difficulty with back pain, I would point to a twisted or rotated spine. Back pain frequently occurs when lifting even minimal weight is done with a twisted posture. When the spine twists, it is at a mechanical disadvantage. The muscles are stretched on one side and short on the other, and, therefore, they are unable to generate the usual support force to the spine. The joints of the back are compressed unnaturally and the added pressure of lifting a weight only causes more damage to the structures.

Rachel, a twenty-two-year-old college student, moved into a fourth-floor apartment in a building without an elevator. She had driven a number of hours, and carrying the furniture up four flights of stairs took the rest of the day. The

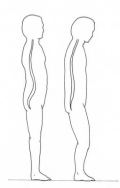

Figure 11.1 Good and poor posture. The left figure has good posture with the head over the pelvis with normal spinal curves. The right figure has poor posture with a flat low back. The flat back causes a forward bend of the knees and neck. This posture fatigues all the muscles of the neck, back, and legs.

mattress was particularly difficult to maneuver, but instead of getting help or pushing the mattress while facing it, Rachel twisted her back to lift it onto the bed. Immediately the injured muscles started to tighten and her range of motion was limited the rest of the day, making the rest of the move very difficult. It took four weeks before the muscle tightness resolved.

Rachel's story highlights the risk associated with bad body mechanics and physical tasks. Think about the way you lift an object *before* you do it, instead of trying to figure out why your back is painful afterward.

Lifting Posture

When lifting any object, your feet and your back should be going in the same direction. You should face the object, bend your hips and knees, and lift with your legs, not your back. The object should be kept as close to your body as possible. If you can, it is better to lift the object from a height as opposed to lifting it from the ground.

If you must lift heavy objects frequently, consider using an abdominal corset to increase intra-abdominal pressure to support your spine. These corsets are not magic—they don't work if they aren't closed around your body. At one of the local hospitals, I noted that many of the hospital employees leave the corsets open. A recent study showed that most people who are given instructions about using abdominal corsets still use them incorrectly. However, the corsets may be helpful, even if left open, if it makes you remember to lift with your legs, not your back.

Standing Posture

Standing in one position for a length of time can lead to fatigued muscles in your lower back. You may have experienced this feeling at a party where no chairs are available, or in a museum with no place to sit down. The upright posture increases the curve in the lumbar spine and stretches the muscle (psoas) in the front of the spine that travels to the hip. Lift one leg to rest on a stool. Transfer weight from foot to foot, or flatten your back with a pelvic tilt (see chapter 8). These positions take pressure off the psoas muscles and the curve of your back. Do these with any activity that requires prolonged standing, such as ironing, giving a lecture, or painting a wall.

Seated Posture

A good sitting posture requires that the height of the seat allows your feet to be flat on the floor, with your knees at slightly above 90 degrees. The back of the chair should support the lumbar curve. Chairs used in offices have an adjustable back and wheels, and the tension and position of the back support should be adjustable along with the height of the seat.

If you are experiencing back pain, the best chair for you has a firm upholstered seat, with a firm straight back and armrests. Wait to use the soft, sofa-type chair when your back pain has totally resolved. In a soft chair, your back is constantly making adjustments to support your spine, and these tiny adjustments can cause fatigue or increase pain because your back is working very hard. When you sit in a chair with firm support, the muscles can relax because the chair supports them.

Stretching Posture

Many of us get into trouble when we stretch. You're the last one on the plane, so you have to stretch to squeeze your carry-on bag into the overhead bin between suitcases that seem to weigh a ton. Or you have to stretch across the bed to tuck a sheet under the corner. Maybe a bag of groceries has shifted to the farthest recesses of your car trunk. In these situations, you may stretch to reach, only to recognize that you are about a foot too short for the task! About five seconds later, the muscles in your low back and side have realized this fact, too, and now they are in spasm.

The simple answer to overstretching is to get closer to the object you want to move. If it is above your head, get a step stool. (If it's in an overhead airline bin, ask for help.) If you must reach the other corner of the bed, put one knee on the mattress and move closer to the corner. Instead of bending over to vacuum, kneel down on your knee to keep your back straight, depending on the type of vacuum you have, of course. Place packages in the front of the trunk, or on the backseat of the car.

Avoid Back Fatigue

Never stay in one position for an extended period of time. Whether you're standing or sitting, change the position and move around at least once an hour, more frequently if your back quickly fatigues. Constant contraction of muscles makes them fatigue, and once that happens, they start to ache. Aching muscles are weaker muscles, and once their functioning is compromised, you are at greater risk for injury.

It's easy to forget simple prevention tips. For example, you may sit like a prisoner on an airplane. But take a stroll to the lavatory even if you don't need it. If you sit at a computer, remind yourself to get up to get your muscles moving. If you spend hours on the phone for your job, get a headset if possible, which allows you to get up and walk around. All these activities improve the function of your lumbar spine, and it will thank you by aching less.

KEEP WORKING

When back pain is related to your job, it is often complicated by the interaction with your employer and the workers' compensation system. And if you were unhappy with your work environment, that could prolong your back pain as well as your return to work. You need to be compensated fairly for loss of working time, and you also need to modify the conditions at your job that caused the back attack in the first place, whether you have a desk job or one that is physically strenuous. It's important to return to work, in any capacity, early in the course of a back attack. The longer you are out of work, the less likely it is that you will ever return to gainful employment. If someone is out of work for one year after a back injury, the chances of returning to a job are essentially zero. Max, a forty-five year-old office worker came to my office three days after the onset of pain associated with a lifting accident at his work. His office was moving to another location in the building, and he had been lifting boxes for two days. He developed pain and stiffness in his back that made it impossible for him to sit at his desk. He had muscle strain associated with lifting (he had twisted his back frequently). He was treated with medications and a five-day sick slip. When he returned to my office, his back pain had improved and his muscle spasm resolved. He was sent back to work with the recommendation that he be excused from any additional lifting associated with his office move. He was encouraged to move frequently during the day. With the modification in his work duties for three weeks, Max had total resolution of his back pain and has returned to his usual job.

The therapies in my basic back pain relief program can help you if you were injured at work. Once you are pain free for five to ten days, returning to work is feasible. Don't carry objects greater than ten pounds initially, even if your job involves heavy lifting. Always use good body mechanics—your feet and face are in line, with no spinal twisting. As you feel more comfortable with lighter lifting tasks, you can progress to lifting heavier objects. If you sit for most of the day, remember that sitting puts strain on the lumbar spine. Get up frequently to relieve back muscle fatigue.

KEEP YOUR BONES STRONG

Starting at an early age, our goal should be to prevent osteoporosis before our bones reach that stage when they weaken and become thin. This means maximizing our bone calcium during adolescence; maintaining bone calcium during adulthood; and for women, minimizing postmenopausal bone loss. Bone calcium increases in children and adolescents who consume higher levels of calcium in food or supplements. However, high calcium intake during the postmenopausal period has no effect—or a minimal protective effect—against bone loss in women. (Men also get osteoporosis, but in smaller numbers.)

To maintain bone strength, most adults should have 1000 to 1500 mg of calcium per day. In addition, regular weight-bearing exercise, like walking, contributes to the development of bone mass, and resistance or impact exercise, such as lifting weights, helps maintain bone mineral levels.

In Caucasian women, calcium intake should be 800 mg a day until age ten, then 1,500 mg during adolescence and pregnancy, and 1,200 mg during adulthood. Vitamin D, 400 to 800 IU, is a valuable supplement used in conjunction with calcium supplements. This is particularly helpful for the elderly who have limited exposure to sunlight, or nutritional deficiency. The combination of these supplements decreases the risk of hip fractures in elderly populations. Non-Caucasian women start with a greater amount of bone mineral calcium. They should take calcium supplements, but they are at less risk for fractures.

Hormone Replacement Therapy for Women

The reason osteoporosis is considered a women's health issue is because estrogen deficiency after menopause leads to bone loss. The greatest rate of bone loss occurs in the first years after cessation of ovarian function. Estrogen replacement therapy, commonly called ERT, is often started soon after the onset of menopause in women who are appropriate candidates. Some women begin hormonal therapy during the perimenopausal periods. ERT is not recommended if you have a history of breast or uterine cancer or clotting disorders. To prevent bone loss with ERT, women need estrogen every day. For women with an intact uterus, progesterone is added because it decreases the risk of uterine cancer. This combination therapy is called HRT, hormone replacement therapy. Controversy remains about the relationship between ERT and breast cancer, and recent epidemiological studies suggest a small association. Using ERT is a personal choice that must be discussed with your physician.

Raloxifene (Evista) is a selective estrogen-receptor modulator (SERM) with estrogenlike effects on bone resorption but without stimulating breast tissue or the lining of the uterus in postmenopausal women. Raloxifene, given in daily doses, effectively increases bone and decreases the risk of spine and hip fracture. Toxic side effects include hot flashes, leg cramps, and rare episodes of venous clotting.

Calcitonin

Calcitonin is a hormone that reduces bone breakdown and is used to treat osteoporosis, and salmon calcitonin is more effective than human calcitonin. Calcitonin is given by injection, or intranasally, on a daily basis. Nasal calcitonin decreases the risk of spinal fractures but may not significantly alter the risk of hip fractures. However, one of the added benefits of calcitonin is its pain-relieving effects, particularly on bone fractures.

Bisphosphonates

Bisphosphonates came into medical use in a roundabout way, and their concept is based on research that studied detergents and hard water. Bisphosphonates attach to bone crystals, the sites of active bone remodeling. Bones are living tissues, constantly being built up and torn down, and bisphosphonates alter bone remodeling by reducing the tearing down portion of remodeling. By decreasing bone resorption, bone density is increased.

Alendronate (Fosamax) effectively prevents and treats osteoporosis because alendronate is a potent inhibiting agent of bone remodeling. Studies of women with established osteoporosis have found that alendronate given every day prevents postmenopausal bone loss and increases bone density in the spine by approximately 4 to 6 percent over a three year period. Alendronate also has a beneficial effect on increasing bone density in the hip. A smaller daily dose of alendronate is comparable to ERT in preventing bone loss. The effect on bone is prolonged, meaning that it's measured in years; therefore, younger women of childbearing years are not candidates for this agent. Alendronate comes in a larger-dose pill that allows administration once a week with the same beneficial effects as the daily dose. The larger dose formulation is more convenient than the smaller daily dose. This weekly regimen decreases exposure of the esophagus and, hence, reduces irritation.

Risedronate (Actonel) decreases the risk of spine and hip fractures as well as increasing bone in these locations. This drug has been recently approved by the FDA for the treatment of postmenopausal osteoporosis at a single daily dose.

The primary toxicity of the bisphosphonates is gastrointestinal, and they tend to have poor intestinal absorption. These drugs must be taken on an empty stomach. For example, alendronate should be taken in the morning after an overnight fast, with a large glass of water. In addition, you should remain upright for thirty minutes to assure that the medication remains out of the esophagus, because heartburn is a common complaint.

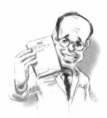

DR. B'S PRESCRIPTION SUMMARY

R℞

- Back pain can be prevented.

- Quit smoking now.

- Maintain general physical fitness.

- Achieve and maintain an appropriate body weight.

- Eat a diet rich in antioxidants and other essential nutrients.

- Utilize good body mechanics to maximize comfortable posture.

- Go back to work once your pain resolves.

- Maintain the strength of your bones with exercise and supplements.

Dr. B—

12

ENJOYING SEX WITHOUT HURTING YOUR BACK

"When can I have sex again?" I wish I heard this question more often, but unfortunately, many men and women are reluctant to ask about sexuality. Perhaps you want to be intimate with your partner but you're worried that the act itself will make your condition worse. Your partner may feel the same way, and he or she may shy away from intimacy with you, with the kindest of intentions. Still, you may see it as rejection. These are the kinds of misunderstandings that can occur when back pain is an issue.

Ignorance and lack of communication lead to misconceptions about sexual health and low back pain. On the other hand, honest, caring discussions, along with psychological support, lead to a strong emotional and sexual bond despite the presence of low back pain. Obviously, the information presented here is not meant to serve as a manual covering all the issues related to sexual health, but rather, it concentrates on helping you remove the barriers that may have formed because of low back pain.

First, the outlook for people with acute low back pain is different from the outlook for chronic pain sufferers. Acute back pain is intense but will resolve, and a short hiatus from sexual activity is easier to tolerate when you expect the problem to resolve. But with chronic back pain you may need to modify sexual activity in order to have a successful relationship.

It's Not All Physical

When no health concerns exist, you and your partner are free to explore a variety of body positions during lovemaking. Spontaneous experimentation may have no consequences other than slight muscle soreness the following day. Under those circumstances, sexual climax may be the measure of a successful interaction. But as we all know, a healthy sexual relationship involves more than physical lovemaking. Sexual intercourse is only a small part of a complex interaction of emotional and physical factors. We sustain partnerships by demonstrating our concern for the other person and by expressing our romantic and affectionate feelings in nonsexual ways, too.

You have a choice when it comes to sex. You can decide that modern society is too caught up with sex, and besides, thanks to media images, only a rare person can reach these ambitious sexual goals. So, you conclude you're better off not worrying about your sexual needs while your back hurts. You can live without sex, so why bother?

Don't give up so fast. A healthy sex life can have beneficial effects on your back pain—and on your general health, too. Sex is a workout for your cardiovascular system, and you also burn a few calories. When you have sex, blood flow increases, which improves the appearance of your skin. Orgasm causes the release of endorphins, chemicals in the brain that act as the body's natural analgesics. Endorphins promote restful sleep and a general sense of well-being. So, indeed, sex is worth the trouble.

If you have acute low back pain, a short respite of a few days may allow your back pain and spasm to improve and sexual movements will not cause increased pain. If you think these sexual motions may increase your discomfort, practice them without your partner. If you don't notice increased discomfort, then sex with your partner is likely to go well. However, if pain occurs with simple movements of the back, wait a bit longer. If your pain is chronic, then you'll need to plan your sexual activity more carefully.

Talk is a Sexy Word

In 1998, in an article published in *Arthritis Today*, Jackson Rainer, Ph.D., said that his favorite four-letter word for intercourse is "talk." Dr. Rainer suggests that romantic interactions can occur when we're sitting together at the kitchen table fully clothed. Of course, the implication is that various levels of communication lay the groundwork for a caring, successful relationship. This is never more important than in the presence of physical limitations. You and your partner need to discuss your respective concerns and ask questions that will lead to greater understanding of the problem you're dealing with. For example:

- What makes your pain worse?
- What activities do not cause pain?
- When is the best time for intimacy?

In addition, both you and your partner may need reassurance about desirability. Do not wait until you are making love to talk about these issues, but instead, plan ahead in order to make the interaction painless and enjoyable. Don't forget romance! Nonphysical interactions support your relationship, and these can include a variety of things from compliments about your partner's appearance to appreciation for his or her emotional support to simple acts that show depth of feelings.

PAINLESS POSITIONS

The best way to find comfortable positions during sex is to recreate the positions that are comfortable to your lower back during everyday activities. For example, if the back support of a particular chair is good, then use that chair for sexual intercourse. Or find the position in bed that causes the least discomfort for your spine. In order to decrease strain on your back, here are some general guidelines:

- Avoid positions that increase the low back curve—that motion causes pressure on the facet joints.
- Avoid lying flat on your stomach.
- Avoid bending forward at the hips with your legs straight—this causes stretching of the sciatic nerve and hamstring muscles.
- Keep the amount of weight your partner puts on your body to a minimum. Place your hands on the bed to support your weight.
- Avoid the man-on-top "missionary position." For men this position increases lumbar lordosis and stretch on low back muscles. For women on the bottom, any movement of the pelvis will require extension of the spine and increased pain.
- The partner without pain should supply the most motion.
- A flat lower back and upward lift to the pelvis (pelvic tilt) is pleasant and protective.

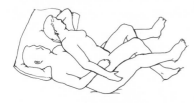

Figure 12.1 Spoon position

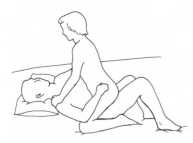

Figure. 12.3 Straddle position

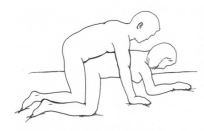

Figure 12.3 All-fours position

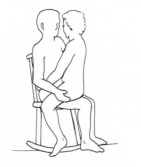

Figure 12.4 Rocking chair

Figures 12.1 through 12.4 show positions that offer maximum comfort during sexual intercourse for men and women. The type of motion matters, too. Rapid thrusts may cause too much discomfort, whereas slow, gradual movements may be less painful and allow for a different sensation than the more athletic activity associated with unrestricted sex. My advice to partners is to tell each other what positions and touches are pleasant and stimulating and to develop signals between you that acknowledge the onset of pain with particular movements.

The spoon position (fig. 12.1) offers the greatest safety for both partners. Pillows strategically placed on the bed can offer correct support to the head, pelvis, and thighs. Both partners have their hips and knees flexed with a pelvic tilt. The flat back protects the facet joints, and the bent hips and knees take the tension off the sciatic nerve and the psoas muscles. Either partner can supply the pelvic movement that offers genital stimulation.

The straddle position (fig. 12.2) may be used with your partner looking toward you or away from you. The partner with back pain should determine the most comfortable position. This position allows your lover's weight to be placed on the bed or your knees (and not your back).

The all-fours position (fig. 12.3) allows sexual intercourse with the partner with back pain to support body weight with the arms. A flexed posture with slow thrusts is possible with this position. If a woman has back pain in this position, it may be best to have a more sturdy foundation on the floor, instead of a bed. With both partners' knees on the floor and a support under the woman's torso, movement of the pelvis will not "rock the boat" and cause involuntary, painful muscle contractions. Speaking of rocking, a rocking chair without arms may offer back support as well as pelvic motion (fig. 12.4). Variations on these themes are allowed as pain decreases.

MEDICATION AND LIBIDO

When low back pain is present, not all sexual difficulties are related to the discomfort itself. Fortunately, erectile dysfunction is rarely related to abnormalities in the lumbar spine, but sometimes the therapies for low back pain may contribute to poor performance. For example, antidepressant medications used for chronic pain as well as depression can cause sexual dysfunction with inhibited ejaculation in men and decreased orgasm in women. Antidepressants can also cause vaginal dryness that results in pain during intercourse. Narcotic medications can decrease pain but also may blunt sexual desire or response, and muscle relaxants may have a similar effect. In addition, excessive alcohol intake is known to suppress libido. Our challenge with medication is to find a balance between a large enough dosage to control pain, and a dose low enough to limit toxicity, including sexual impairment.

Fatigue interferes with successful sexual performance, and fatigue only amplifies pain. The old adage "plan ahead" certainly applies to eliminating fatigue. If you desire a successful sexual encounter, then make sure you're well rested.

Sexual Satisfaction at Sixty

Tom, age sixty, had low back pain from osteoarthritis of the spine. After six months of treatment, his pain had improved but not enough for him to continue a satisfactory sexual relationship with his wife. The missionary position was particularly bothersome. He had been doing flexion exercises earlier in his treatment, but he had stopped them a few months before I saw him. He was taking Oruvail (ketoprofen) in a sustained-release form for his pain. I suggested an additional dose of ketoprofen or acetaminophen prior to sexual activity, and I suggested alternative sexual positions. This combination proved successful, and eighteen months after my recommendations, his low back pain was improving and his sexual function is better as well.

Tom's case illustrates that sexual performance can benefit from careful timing of medication. To allow for adequate analgesia, take your pain medication two to four hours before planned sexual activity.

If sexual climax cannot be achieved through intercourse, then you and your partner should discuss alternative techniques. This may be difficult if there are social, cultural, or spiritual barriers to oral sexual stimulation, but I recommend discussing these issues because situations exist in which back pain limits the ability to engage in sexual intercourse. In addition, those with increased tension in sex organs that prevents orgasm through other means should consider self-stimulation. Releasing sexual tension by any of these means decreases muscle contraction and increases endorphin levels.

SEXERCISES

Exercise helps improve sexual satisfaction, and any form of aerobic exercise improves cardiovascular function and increases stamina. In particular, Kegel exercises for the pelvis increase sexual enjoyment for women by strengthening the pelvic floor muscles supporting the bladder, uterus, rectum, and vagina. These are the muscles that contract around the penis during intercourse.

Kegel exercises are easily performed while urinating. Slowly contract the pelvic floor muscles, a motion that halts urine flow. Hold the contraction for ten seconds, release, and repeat the contraction several times. The same muscles can be contracted at other times while standing, sitting, or lying down. Do twenty-five to fifty contractions twice a day.

Additional Consultation

If you continue to have sexual difficulties beyond that of back pain alone, consider seeking help from a sex therapist or a psychiatrist. Back pain is sometimes used as an excuse for limiting sexual relationships. Or, if your relationship is already troubled, then back pain may further complicate your problems. Simply changing your sexual position is not enough to change feelings, and a solution can be found only through improved communication. Consider additional help if necessary, but do not let your relationship deteriorate.

A healthy and understanding sexual relationship is a part of the complete prescription for a better back. You do not have to forgo the pleasures of this human interaction just because you have back pain. The benefits are worth the effort.

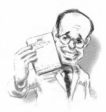

DR. B'S PRESCRIPTION SUMMARY

R

- Back pain should never prevent you from having a successful sexual relationship.

- Sexual intimacy has multiple health benefits.

- "Talk" is a sexy four-letter word.

- Practice the most painless sexual positions, such as keeping your back flat, and avoiding the missionary position, which increases the curve to your lower back.

- Talk with your doctor about your medications if you think they are limiting your sexual performance.

Dr. B—

EPILOGUE

BACK IN CONTROL!

You should now have a good idea how to put together the parts of your prescription that will work for you. I have mentioned a wide range of therapies that are effective for low back pain. I prefer active therapies to passive ones. That is my bias. Active therapies leave you in charge so you can control your recovery—back in control. That is also why I prefer conventional therapies over complementary. Many complementary therapies, in addition to being time consuming, require the intervention of others.

Currently, research signals great hope for major advances in prevention, diagnosis, and treatment of back pain. Genetics research will help us understand hereditary factors that predispose to the development of disc degeneration. We will identify environmental factors that cause disc degeneration so we can prevent it. More sensitive diagnostic tests will allow us to visualize the spine in motion and see injured muscles clearly. More effective and less toxic NSAIDs are on the horizon. The second generation of COX-2 inhibitors is now in clinical trials, and new muscle relaxants are also being developed. Artificial disc replacements are being tested, and new fusion techniques won't require taking bone from the pelvis. The increasing interest in occupational therapy is shedding new light on ergonomic factors that limit the risk for back pain at the workplace. The future will improve our understanding of the factors that cause back pain. Our ability to take care of the persons with back pain will also improve.

Until that time, educate yourself about your back. Being educated will promote your improvement and save you exposure to diagnostic tests or therapeutic interventions that can have more risks than benefits. Use your knowledge with your primary care physician, with your physical therapist, with your anesthesiologist, with your massage therapist. Ask questions. Be critical of the answers. Decide what makes the most sense to you. Be back in control!

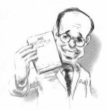

DR. B'S PRESCRIPTION SUMMARY

R

- Be active in your recovery.

- Be informed.

- Keep moving.

- Use medicines as needed.

- Do exercises to remain strong.

Dr. B—

GLOSSARY

ACUPUNTURE: The Chinese practice of stimulating particular locations along the body's meridians to free the flow of energy (*qi*).

ANALGESICS: Medications that relieve pain like nonsteroidals (aspirin), nonnarcotics (acetaminophen), or narcotics (codeine).

ANKYLOSING SPONDLITIS (AS): An inflammatory arthritis of the spine associated with pain and stiffness that can result in the fusion (ankylosis) of the spinal joints and ligaments.

ANNULUS FIBROSUS: The circular outer portion of the intervertebral disc.

ANTI-INFLAMMATORY: Reducing heat, swelling, pain, and loss of function.

ARACHNOIDITIS: Inflammation of the membrane surrounding the spinal cord.

ARTHRITIS: Inflammation of a joint.

CAUDA EQUINA: The end of the spinal cord that starts at L-1 and resembles the "tail of a horse."

CERVICAL: Relating to the seven vertebrae in the neck between the skull and chest.

COCCYX: The end of the spine, the tailbone. It is connected to the sacrum.

COMPUTED TOMOGRAPHY (CT): A radiographic technique utilizing X rays and computer technology to visualize horizontal sections of the human body. Most useful for identifying bone abnormalities.

CONJUNCTIVITIS: Inflammation of the superficial layer of the eye.

CONVERSION REACTION: Transformation of an emotion into a physical manifestation, hysteria.

CORTICOSTEROIDS: Hormones produced by the adrenal gland with properties to influence glucose metabolism and kidney function. A decrease in inflammation is a potential result of ingesting amounts greater than those produced by the adrenal gland on a daily basis.

CYCLOOXYGENASE: An enzyme that comes in two forms, I and II. Type I maintains body functions. Type II is associated with the development of inflammation. Aspirin inhibits I and II. COX-2 drugs inhibit Type II only.

DEGENERATION: A deterioration of tissues and cells that results in impairment or destruction of the structure.

DISC: The cylinder-like structure composed of a gel center (nucleus pulposus) and a fibrous outer covering (annulus fibrosus) that acts as a shock absorber and a universal joint in the spine.

DISCECTOMY: Removal of all or part of an intervertebral disc.

DISCOGRAPHY: Radiographic visualization of the intervertebral disc space by injection of dye.

ERGONOMICS: The scientific study of the efficient use of the human body in work and recreation.

EXTENSION: In regard to the spine, bending backward.

FACET JOINTS: The paired joints located in the posterior portion of the vertebral bodies connecting the spine. These joints are part of the stabilizing mechanism for the spine.

FASCIA: A thin sheet of fibrous tissue enveloping muscles and structures below the skin.

Glossary

FIBROMYALGIA: A generalized musculoskeletal syndrome associated with tender points in specific locations on the body.

FLEXION: In regard to the spine, bending forward.

FUSION: In regard to the spine, a surgical procedure to unite two or more vertebrae with bone graft with or without metal supports resulting in immobilization of that portion.

GADOLINIUM: The contrast material utilized with magnetic resonance imaging (MRI) to identify tissues with increased blood flow. Used to identify tumors, postsurgical scar tissue, and infections.

GENE: The unit of a chromosome that transfers an inherited characteristic from parent to offspring.

HAMSTRING: The muscles and tendons located in the back of the thigh.

HERNIATED DISC: Displacement of the central portion of an intervertebral disc (nucleus pulposus). The degrees of herniation include protrusion (gel contained within the annulus fibrosis), extrusion (gel displaced into the spinal canal beyond the annulus but remains connected to the central area), and sequestration (gel free and unattached to the original disc).

INFLAMMATION: A pathologic process associated with redness, heat, swelling, pain, and loss of function. This process destroys tissues but is also associated with the repair and healing of body structures.

INTERVERTEBRAL: Between two adjacent vertebrae.

JOINT: A specialized structure where two bones come in close proximity. The joint may facilitate movement (facet) or stability (sacroiliac) depending on the function of the joint.

KYPHOSIS: A deformity of the spine associated with excessive forward bending, most commonly in the thoracic area.

LAMINECTOMY: A surgical procedure that removes a portion of the plate that serves as the back of the spinal canal. This decompression procedure is performed for treatment of herniated intervertebral discs and spinal stenosis.

LIGAMENT: A strong band of fibrous tissue connecting bones at a joint or holding organs in place.

LORDOSIS: The forward curve located in the low back and neck.

LOW BACK: The area between the lower ribs and the lower crease of the buttocks.

LUMBAR: Relating to the five vertebrae between the chest and sacrum.

MAGNETIC RESONANCE IMAGING (MRI): A radiographic technique utilizing magnets and radio waves to visualize the internal structures of the human body. Overall, the most useful technique in the investigation of spinal abnormalities.

MANIPULATION: Movement of the spine to restore normal function.

MUSCLE: Specialized contractile tissue that generates force and facilitates movement.

MYELOGRAM: A radiographic technique where dye is injected into the spinal canal to better identify the spinal cord.

NARCOTIC: A powerful pain-relieving drug associated with potential to cause significant alteration of mood and dependence following repeated administration.

NERVE: Specialized cordlike tissue that transmits signals to and from the brain.

NONSTEROIDAL: A medication that decreases inflammation that is not a corticosteroid.

NUCLEUS PULPOSUS: The gel center of the intervertebral disc. This is the portion of the disc that herniates.

OSTEOARTHRITIS: The most common form of arthritis. The lumbar spine is a frequent location for this disorder.

OSTEOPOROSIS: A disorder associated with decreased calcium in bone. This disorder is associated with increased risk of fracture in the spine, hip, and wrist.

Glossary

PLACEBO: An inert substance that is used in medical research to determine the degree of improvement that occurs by chance alone.

RAD: A measure of radiation exposure. Normal background exposure to the sun during a year is about 0.6 rads.

RADIONUCLIDE SCAN: A radiographic test using a small amount of radioactive tracer that is injected intravenously. The tracer identifies tissues with abnormally increased activity. A bone scan is the test most frequently used to survey the entire spine for low back disorders.

RADICULOPATHY: A disorder of the nerves after they exit the spine.

REFLEX: An involuntary action that results from sensory input causing a muscular response.

REITER'S SYNDROME: A disorder that causes conjunctivitis, urethritis, and arthritis. The lumbar spine and sacroiliac joints are injured in this disease.

RHEUMATISM: Any ache or pain in the musculoskeletal system. Arthritis is a special form of rheumatism.

SACRUM: Relating to the portion of the spine between the lumbar and coccyx. The sacroiliac joints connect the sacrum with the pelvis.

SCIATICA: A pain that follows the sciatic nerve down the leg to the calf or foot.

SCOLIOSIS: A lateral curvature of the spine.

SPINAL CORD: The major nerve structure located within the spine that connects the brain with the rest of the human body.

SPONDYLOARTHROPATHY: A group of disorders that causes inflammatory arthritis of the spine.

SPONDYLOLISTHESIS: An anterior displacement of a vertebra on the one below that can be the result of a spondylolysis that occurred during development as a teenager, or through degenerative changes in the facet joints.

SPONDYLOLYSIS: A defect in the growth plate between the joints in the back of a vertebra.

SPONDYLOSIS: A degenerative disease of the discs and facet joints of the spine.

STRAIN: An injury that occurs from overuse, frequently associated with muscles, fascia, and ligaments.

SUBLUXATION: An abnormal movement or position of joint surfaces.

SYNDROME: A collection of complaints that together describe a disorder.

TENDON: A tough, fibrous structure that attaches muscles to bones.

URETHRITIS: Inflammation of the lining of the urethra, the tube that connects the bladder with the surface of the body.

VERTEBRA: One of the individual bones that form the spine. The shape and function of the vertebrae are specific to the different portions of the spine.

X RAYS: A form of electromagnetic energy that passes through an object, forming a charged particle that is imaged on a piece of film.

APPENDIX A

DR. B'S
BACK SCHOOL FAQ

In the late 1960s, a Swedish physical therapist, Maryanne Zachrisson-Forssell, developed a sound-slide program that included basic information about low back pain. The four one-hour sessions included information of anatomy and function of the spine, body mechanics, and exercise programs. The classes also included question-and-answer sessions to address any issues that were not addressed during the slide lectures.

The enthusiasm for back schools in the United States slowly increased over time. Physicians, physical therapists, and nurse specialists teach the courses. Back schools exist in medical schools, community hospitals, YMCAs, and industrial settings.

The methods of teaching vary at back school depending on the philosophy of the organizers. "Students" may be given classroom instruction, or demonstrations of exercises and work habits, or motivation. Teaching methods vary around the world. The Swedish Back School is designed as a general information program with an exercise program to improve physical conditioning. The Canadian Back School uses psychological approaches to increase self-awareness about pain and function. The role of anxiety and stress is emphasized. The California Back School teaches how to control acute low back pain. Individuals go through an obstacle course to measure physical function. Instruction over a three-week period improves physical function.

Do back schools help people prevent recurrences of back pain? A study was conducted in a Volvo car plant where back school instruction was matched against back exercises or heat therapy. Employees who attended back school had fewer days off work than the other two groups.

When I was the director of the Spine Center at the local medical center, I helped organize their back school. A number of back pain sufferers became students at the school. The instructors of the classes had an opportunity to compile a number of questions that were repeatedly asked at the back school sessions. Here are some of the most frequently asked questions and my most current answers.

What kind of bed is best for back pain?

You would think that with as much time as people have been sleeping on beds I would have the answer to this question. What seems to be clear is that preferences are as numerous as the people who go to sleep every night.

When I began my professional career, I thought only a rock-hard bed would be best for back pain patients. Over the years, I have learned that what may be good for a person on one side of the bed may not be so good for the other. How do you solve this dilemma?

There are a few ways of testing what makes your back better before buying a bed. The back, between the pelvis and the shoulders, is like an upside-down suspension bridge. The supports for this semicircle are the buttocks and shoulders. The firmer the bed, the more the supports will stay above the water and keep tension in the back, maintaining the lumbar curve, or lordosis. The softer the bed, the more the supports will sink, placing less tension on the lumbar spine, causing it to lose the lordosis, or flatten.

The more you want to maintain a lumbar curve, the firmer the mattress you want. If you want to test this idea, try sleeping on a few blankets or an exercise mat on the floor for a few nights. If your back feels rested, a hard mattress is for you. If you prefer a flat back, a softer mattress will do.

Another way to test this idea is by testing what effect the position of your legs has on your pain. If you prefer to have your legs flat on the bed, you will prefer a hard mattress. If you prefer your knees bent, you will prefer a mattress with more padding.

These suggestions are starting points to decide on your personal preference. You will be sleeping on the bed and need to decide if it will be restful to you. Do not be bashful. Go to the mattress store and test out the merchandise. Rest on them for twenty to thirty minutes to feel if they are comfortable. Having some medical name (chiropractic, orthopaedic) associated with the name of the bed does not guarantee that the bed will be good for you. The only way to know is to test it out.

I love to swim, but making waves at night was never one of my ideas of how to sleep. Despite my apprehensions about waterbeds, some back pain sufferers swear by them. I do not know how that degree of softness can be helpful to the spine. I believe that, given the choice, those who prefer a flat back will prefer a waterbed. Once again, try it out before you buy one.

Some mattresses are reported to contour specifically to your body and support your back no matter what its shape. These mattresses use special foam or air to support the back. Some of my patients have found these to be excellent, while others have found them less desirable. The idea of full support is a good one, but some patients require a firmer surface for comfort.

What happens if you have a bed already and you do not want to purchase a new one? A bed can be made firmer by placing a piece of plywood between the mattress and box spring. If you have to make a bed softer, adding cushioning in the form of a mattress pad can be effective.

Is any particular chair helpful for low back pain?

It depends on the location of the chair: at work, at home, or in the car. Is the chair to prevent pain or to treat pain? There's no one chair for all locations and situations.

In the acute low back pain situation, the very stable, firm chair is best. The chair should have a small amount of cushioning for comfort. The area on the surface of the seat should allow some movement of the legs. The chair seat should not be too low, causing your legs to be close to your chest. Legs should be at ninety degrees or slightly higher than your hips if you prefer a flat back. The back of the chair should have a slight angle. Armrests decrease pressure on your low back.

A variety of lumbar lordosis seat supports are available. Some pillows are made of foam, while some are inflatable. See if you would benefit from a seat support by rolling up a towel and putting it around your waist. If the addition of the towel decreases your pain, you should consider a seat support. The support can be used on the chair at work and in the car.

Designers of new car models realize the importance of seat supports and have built in adjustments into the seat in the car that can be altered for comfort. Do not be afraid to try different positions of the seat to try to maximize comfort. Other car seats are too soft for comfort when you have back pain. The lack of support makes the muscles of the back work constantly, causing increased spasm and pain. A support for the back of the car seat may be adequate if the seat bottom offers adequate stability. If the seat is too soft, a single support that includes a seat bottom and back is useful.

A number of recliners are available with a variety of adjustments for comfort. I believe these chairs to be more comfortable when you are rehabilitating from your back attack as opposed to being in the middle of one. The amount of cushioning, the degree of reclining, and massage and heat attachments are matters of personal preference. None of these factors are particularly helpful in preventing back pain. If they make you feel better and the price is in your budget, you should pamper yourself.

When talking about the office, not all your work has to be done while you are seated. In fact, for some people with leg pain, a standing work desk can offer comfort at work. A forty-eight-year-old attorney came to my office because of increasing pain while at work. He'd had a cervical and lumbar spine operation within the last four years, and he had a recurrence of leg pain that was responding to conservative management. His greatest problem was long hours at work and during conferences. He had tried a number of chairs, but none would allow him to work for any length of time. I suggested that he obtain a standing work desk and use that whenever his leg became painful. I also suggested that he stand more at conferences. The combination helped calm his leg pain over the next six months. He became so fond of his standing desk that he kept on using it even after his leg pain resolved.

The bottom line is try out any seat, recliner, cushion, massager, corset, or support before you make a purchase, do not go by reputation alone.

Do children get back pain?

Back pain does affect children, but less frequently than adults. Young children under ten get back pain infrequently, but in adolescence, from fifteen on, it occurs more frequently. If back pain persists in a child more than one or two weeks, a doctor should evaluate the child. Most back pain in children is mechanical, just like it is in adults. Spondylolysis and spondylolisthesis are fractures of the back of the vertebral body and start during teenage years, particularly in divers and gymnasts. Disc herniations are extremely rare.

Systemic illnesses, such as infections and tumors, do occur in children but are unusual. The red flags for more serious illnesses are the same for adults and children.

A current problem affecting children of all ages is what they are wearing on their backs. More and more kids of school age are having back problems because of heavy backpacks and book bags. These heavy bags strain the muscles of the back and cause fatigue that aches. You can see some kids waiting at the bus stop bent over from the weight on their backs. Book bags should not weigh more than 10 percent to 15 percent of the child's weight. If they are too heavy, lighten them up. The bag should have adjustable straps. The bag should be worn over both shoulders. The shoulders should carry most of the weight. Bags hanging too high or too low on the back place strain across the lumbar spine, causing low back pain.

Does lumbar traction help back pain?

Traction has not been shown to be helpful for low back or leg pain. Traction used to be a way to get patients to stay in bed in the hospital. But we know now that bed rest for longer than two days is not helpful for low back pain. Traction of the lumbar spine is not a recommended therapy. It does nothing for relieving pressure on a disc and places you at risk for the consequences of prolonged bed rest.

Do my high heel shoes cause more back pain?

Sometimes. High heel shoes raise you off the ground, tending to shift your center of gravity. In response to this new position, you may bend backward to stay in balance. The higher the heel, the greater is the apparent sway in the back. If bending backward on dry land makes your back feel worse, so will high heels. A compromise may be shoes that are between flats and full high heels. They do not cause as much of a change in the shape of the spine and may be acceptable from a fashion point of view. The other possibility when wearing a higher heel is limiting the time you stand in them and doing pelvic tilt exercises to flatten your spine when the opportunity allows.

What does that circular mean that comes with my prescription drug package? It scares me half to death.

The package circular is the information supplied by the drug manufacturer that is required by the FDA. It contains basic information about the drug, including all the possible side effects and drug interactions.

The information regarding the *potential* side effects of a drug is generated during the clinical trials studying the efficacy of the agent. As a clinical investigator, I have had personal experience with the information gathered during these trials. If any change occurs during the study, that information is considered an adverse event. This information is counted during the study and the final number is listed in the package circular.

Anything is possible, but the side effects that occur frequently are really the only ones to be concerned about. For example, in one package circular that I reviewed, food poisoning was listed as a possible side effect. Obviously, someone taking part in the study went to a restaurant and had a bad meal. Even though that had nothing to do with the study drug, that happening was considered an adverse event. This kind of information dilutes the value of this important source of information for patients and doctors.

Remember the package circular lists problems that *may* happen. You may experience none of them. However, if you become aware of some interaction, tell your doctor immediately, so he or she can decide if the medicine is the best one to improve your condition.

What sports can I safely play if I have back pain?

In the acute stage of back pain, limiting sports activities is appropriate. Movement is important, but shooting eighteen holes is not going to be helpful. Allowing your back to heal will actually allow you to return and stay functional as opposed to going back too soon and having recurrent attacks stretching out your recovery.

Sport activities can be divided into low, moderate, and high risk for developing low back pain. If you have back pain and are trying to start a new sport, you should speak with your physician before starting a new activity. In general, some of the low-risk sports are compatible with low back pain. These sports are bicycling and swimming. Racquet sports are difficult to start if you are having acute back pain. Also, I have assumed that amateur sports persons are involved with these activities. Professional athletes have greater risks.

- Low-risk sports: bicycling, hockey, skiing, soccer, squash, swimming, tennis
- Moderate-risk sports: baseball, basketball, bowling, some types of dancing, golf, horseback riding, jogging, rowing
- High-risk sports: diving, football, gymnastics, weight lifting

The low-risk sports in general put little pressure on the spine. In addition, the risk of continuous twisting is small. The moderate-risk sports are associated with jumping (basketball, dancing, horseback riding, jogging) or twisting (baseball, bowling, golf, rowing). Jumping places increased pressures on discs. Discs are at risk of herniation or more rapid degeneration. Twisting places pressure on the facet joints. Continuous twisting causes increased joint pain that continues after the sports activity is completed. High-risk sports are associated with high velocity impact (diving, football) or hyperextension (gymnastics) or excessive weight (lifting).

General recommendations for all sports are to use good technique from the outset. You should learn from a good teacher if you have not had experience with the sport. You should ask a ski instructor about appropriate technique to protect your back. You should use appropriate equipment to decrease your exposure to risk. For example, good running shoes with appropriate cushioning are important. Running on soft surfaces like grass or asphalt is better than running on concrete.

Can I play golf without increasing my back pain?

Low back pain problems are the most frequent injury in amateur golfers. This problem also occurs frequently in professional golfers. Golf injuries occur from overuse and develop over time. Amateur golfers are at risk because they play sporadically, without proper warm-up, and have less-than-ideal swing mechanics. Overpracticing poor mechanics increases the risk of injury.

The golf swing results in the riskiest motions for your spine—a hyperextension and rotation. Back pain results from the rotation of the spine in the back swing, and hyperextension in the follow-through. These motions place many times the golfer's body weight across the lower discs of the lumbar spine.

Back problems can be prevented if appropriate care is given to preparation and appropriate technique. It is imperative that golfers warm up for at least ten minutes and include the following:

Stretching (two minutes)
• Neck rotations
• Shoulder stretch
• Trunk side bends
• Trunk rotation
• Toe touches (sitting on bench)

Driving range (three minutes)
• Half swing—sand wedge
• Three-quarter swing—5 iron
• Full swing—driver

Putting (four minutes)
• Back-and-forth putting green
• Waiting to tee off (one minute)
• Practice swings
• Visualize good form

When in doubt, consider lessons from the golf professional to perfect your swing. Appropriate warm-up and good technique are the best ways to decrease overrotation and hyperextension that increase the risk for low back injuries.

APPENDIX B

MEDICATIONS FOR LOW BACK PAIN

Trade Name (Chemical Class)	Dosage (mg)	Frequency (times/day)	Half-life (hours)	Comment
NSAIDs				
Anaprox (naproxen sodium)	275/550	3–4	13	OTC brand is Aleve
Ansaid (flurbiprofen)	50/100	2–3	6	long-acting ibuprofen
Arthrotec (diclofenac/misoprostil)	50/75	2–3	2	prevents stomach ulcers
Ascriptin (aspirin + antacid)	325	4–6	4	
Bayer (aspirin)	325	4–6	4	inexpensive
Cataflam (diclofenac potassium)	25/50	2–3	2	rapid onset of action
Celebrex (celecoxib)	100/200	2	11	less risk of ulcers (Cox-2)
Clinoril (sulindac)	150/200	2	18	
Daypro (oxaprozin)	600	1–2	25	once a day convenience
Disalcid (salsalate)	500/750	2	4	
Dolobid (diflunisal)	250/500	2–3	11	
Easpirin (enteric-coated aspirin)	975	4	4	less GI upset
Ecotrin (enteric-coated aspirin)	325	4–6	4	less GI upset
Feldene (piroxicam)	10/20	1	38–45	long-acting
Indocin (indomethacin)	50–100	1–3	4	for spondyloarthropathy
Lodine (etodalac)	200–500	2–4	6	
Meclomen (meclofenemate)	50/100	4	4	
Mobic (meloxicam)	7.5/15	1	15	like Cox-2 drug
Motrin (ibuprofen)	400–800	4–6	1–3	requires large doses
Nalfon (fenoprofen)	200/300	3–4	2–3	more kidney irritation
Naprelan (naproxen)	375/500	2–3	13	OTC brand is Aleve
Orudis (ketoprofen)	25–75	3–4	3–4	
Oruvail (ketoprofen)	100–200	1	3–4	extended release form
Relafen (nabumetone)	500/750	2	2–6	less GI distress
Tolectin (tolmetin)	200/400	4	4	
Toradol (kerotolac)	10	4	4–6	analgesic, but ulcer risk
Trilisate (choline magnesium trisaliclate)	500/750	2	4	
Vioxx (rofecoxib)	12.5–50	1	18	less risk of ulcers (Cox-2)
Volatren (diclofenac sodium)	25–100	2–3	2	
Zorprin (time-release aspirin)	800	2	4	less GI upse

Back in Control!

Trade Name (Chemical Class)	Dosage (mg)	Frequency (times/day)	Half-life (hours)	Comment
NON-NARCOTIC ANALGESICS				
Tylenol (acetaminophen)	325–650	3	4	no alcohol intake
Ultram (tramadol)	50	4	4	requires frequent doses
NARCOTIC ANALGESICS				
Codeine (codeine)	15–60	4–6	4	
Darvocet (propoxyphene/acetaminophen)	50	4	4	
Darvon (propoxyphene)	65	4	4	
Darvon Compound (propoxyphene/aspirin)	50	4	4	
Darvon-N (propoxyphene)	100	4	4	
Duragesic (fentanyl)	25–100	1	72	topical (on skin)
Kadian (morphine)	20–100	1	12	
Lortab (hydrocodone/acetaminophen)	2.5–10	4	4	
MS Contin (morphine)	15–200	2	12	
Oxycontin (oxycodone)	10–160	2	12	long-acting, less euphoria
Percocet (oxycodone/acetaminophen)	2.5–10	4	4	
Percodan (oxycodone/aspirin)	4.5	4	4	
Tylenol #2/3/4 (codeine/acetaminophen)	15–60	4	4	
Vicodin (hydrocodone/acetaminophen)	5–10	4	4	
Vicoprofen (hydrocodone/ibuprofen)	7.5	4	4	
MUSCLE RELAXANTS				
Flexaril (cyclobenzaprine)	10	2	24–72	sleepiness a toxicity
Norflex (ophenadrine)	100	4	2	
Parafon (chlorzoxazone)	500	4–6	4	
Robaxin (methocarbamol)	500/750	4	2	
Skelaxin (metcaxalone)	400	4	3	
Soma (carisoprodol)	350	4	4–6	addictive properties
Valium (diazepam)	2/5/10	4	24	withdrawal problems
Zanaflex (tizanidine)	4	3	8	

APPENDIX C

BEST BACK RESOURCES

Back in Control
Website: www.backincontrol.net
This website contains references for this book. Updated information on FAQ and patient profiles added on a regular basis.

American College of Rheumatology (ACR)
1800 Century Place, Suite 250
Atlanta, GA 30345-4300
Phone: (404) 633-3777
Website: www.rheumatology.org
The national professional organization of rheumatologists

Arthritis Foundation (AF)
1330 West Peachtree Street
Atlanta, GA 30309
Website: www.arthritis.org
The national organization for the support of individuals with all forms of arthritis

American Academy of Orthopedic Surgeons (AAOS)
6300 N. River Road
Rosemont, IL 60018-4262
Phone: (800) 346-2267
Website: www.aaos.org
The national professional organization of orthopedic surgeons

American Osteopathic Association
142 East Ontario Street
Chicago, IL 60611
Phone: (800) 621-1773
Website: www.am-osteo-assn.org
The national professional organization of osteopathic physicians

American Physical Therapy Association (APTA)
111 North Fairfax Street
Alexandria, VA 22314
Phone: (800) 999-2782
Website: www.apta.org
The national professional organization for physical therapists

American Chiropractic Association
1701 Clarendon Boulevard
Arlington, VA 22209
Phone: (800) 986-4636
Website: www.amerchiro.org
The national professional organization of chiropractors

American Massage Therapy Association
820 David Street, Suite 100
Evanston, IL 60201
Phone: (847) 864-0123
Website: www.amtamassage.org
The national professional organization for massage therapists

National Library of Medicine
Website: www.nlm.nih.gov

National Institutes of Health
Bethesda, MD 20892
Phone: (301) 496-4000
Website: www.nih.gov

National Center for Complementary and Alternative Medicine
Website: www.nccam.nih.gov

Agency for Health Care Policy and Research (AHCPR)

Website: www.ahcpr.gov
Food and Drug Administration
Website: www.fda.gov

Spondylitis Association of America
P.O. Box 5872
Sherman Oaks, CA 91413
Phone: (800) 777-8189
Website: www.spondylitis.org

National Center for Homeopathy
801 North Fairfax Street, Suite 306
Alexandria, VA 22314
Phone: (703) 548-7790
Website: www.healthy.net/nch/

The Pilates Method
Website: www.pilates_studio.com

Inclusion of Web sites or other publications in this appendix does not imply approval of their content.

Other Helpful Publications

Bigos, S. J., O. Bowyer, G. Braen, et al. *Acute Low Back Problems in Adults.* Clinical Practice Guideline No.14. AHCPR Publication No. 95-0642. Rockville, MD: Agency for Health Care Policy and Research, Public Health Service, U.S. Department of Health and Human Services, December 1994, pp. 160.

Borenstein D. G., S. W. Wiesel, S. D. Boden. *Low Back Pain: Medical Diagnosis and Comprehensive Management.* Philadelphia: W. B. Saunders, 1995.

Horstman, J. *The Arthritis Foundation's Guide to Alternative Therapies.* Atlanta: Arthritis Foundation, 1999.

Jellin J. M. (ed). *Natural Medicine: Comprehensive Database.* Stockton: Therapeutic Research Faculty, 1999, pp. 1164.

Rybacki J. J., J. W. Long. *The Essential Guide to Prescription Drugs.* 2001 edition. New York: HarperCollins, 2001, pp. 1274.

INDEX

Index

Index

ABOUT THE AUTHOR

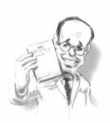 David Borenstein, M.D., is clinical professor of medicine and former medical director of the Spine Center and the George Washington University Medical Center. Dr. Borenstein is a board-certified internist and rheumatologist who is internationally recognized for his expertise in the care of patients with back pain and spinal disorders. Dr. Borenstein received his undergraduate degree from Columbia University in 1969. His medical school, internal medicine residency, and rheumatology fellowship training were completed at the Johns Hopkins University Medical School and Hospital from 1969 to 1978. he became an assistant professor of medicine at the George Washington University Medical Center in 1978. He was promoted to professor of medicine in 1989. He became a clinical professor of medicine on the voluntary faculty in 1997.

Dr. Borenstein is an author of a number of medical articles and books, including *Low Back Pain: Medical Diagnosis and Comprehensive Management (2nd ed.)*. This book has been recognized by the Medical Library Association Brandon/Hill list as one of the 200 essential books for a medical library. He is also author of *Neck Pain: Medical Diagnosis and Management*. He has lectured to the general public on behalf of the Arthritis Foundation on a wide variety of medical topics. He has chaired low back pain symposia for a number of physician groups, including the American College of Rheumatology. He has also moderated national telesymposia sponsored by pharmaceutical companies for physicians. He has also served as a medical guest expert for CNN and local news programs.

Dr. Borenstein is a fellow of the American College of Physicians and American College of Rheumatology. He is a member of the International Society for the Study of the Lumbar Spine and is listed in The Best Doctors in America, Year 200 Edition. He is included in *Who's Who in Medicine and Healthcare, 2nd edition* and *Who's Who in America, 54th edition*. He is in active clinical practice in Washington, D.C.